Gastric Sleeve Bariatric Diet Cookbook

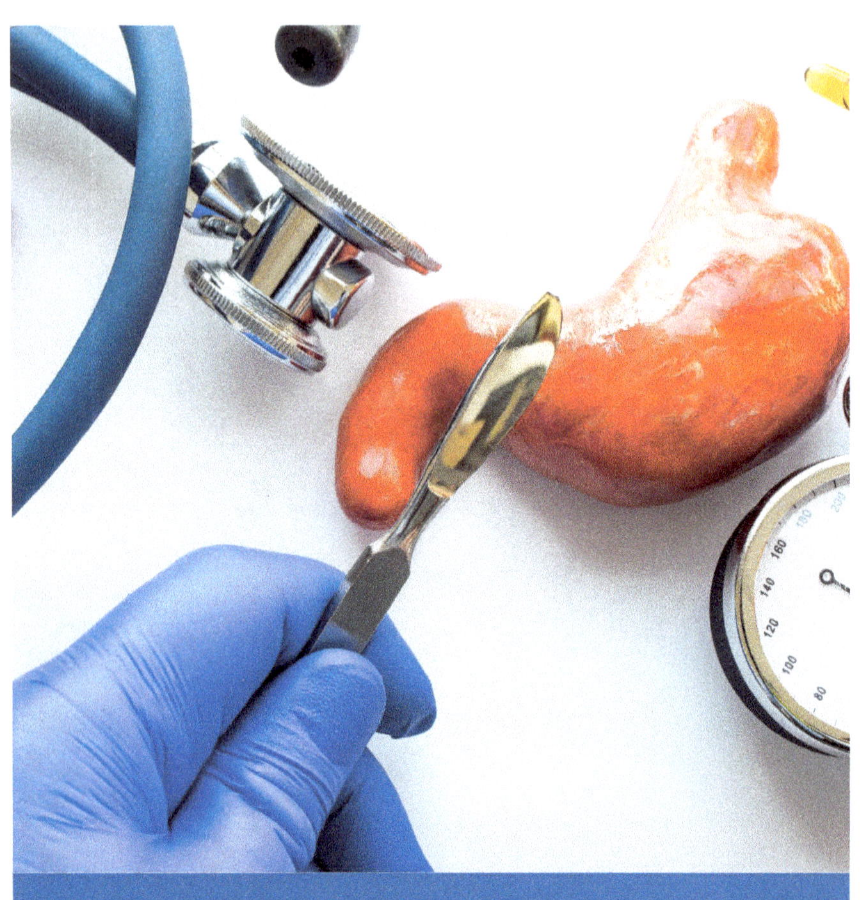

100+ EASY AND SIMPLE PRE-OP AND POST-OP BARIATRIC COOKBOOK FOR GASTRIC BYPASS AND QUICK RECOVERY

This book is dedicated to all the bariatric patients who have started along this path to a better and happier life. Your fortitude, tenacity, and dedication to maintaining your health serve as an example to us all.

ACKNOWLEDGMENTS

The medical experts, dietitians, and chefs who have lent their knowledge and enthusiasm to this book deserve our sincere appreciation. Your advice and suggestions were really helpful in developing a tool that would aid bariatric patients in achieving their wellness and health objectives.

We also want to express our gratitude to our families, friends, and other loved ones for their constant support and inspiration throughout this effort. We have never stopped being inspired and driven by your love and believe in us.

TABLE OF CONTENT

INTRODUCTION

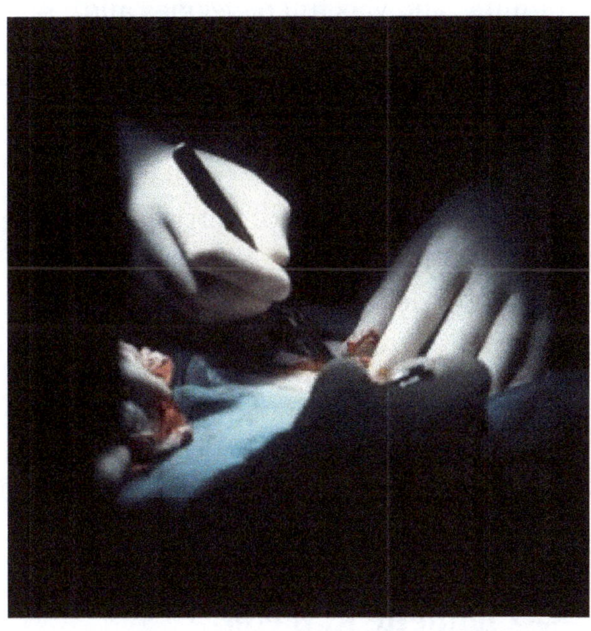 For some who have battled obesity for the majority of their life, losing weight may be a challenging process. I was eager to begin my weight reduction journey and finally reach my health objectives when I had gastric sleeve surgery. But still I quickly understood that eating a good, balanced diet was essential for my

performance. The Gastric Sleeve Bariatric Diet Cookbook came into my possession at that time, and it completely turned my life around. This cookbook saved my life and enabled me to maintain my healthy eating routine.

The cookbook is brimming with delicious and healthful dishes created especially for those who have had gastric sleeve surgery. Each dish has a high protein content, is low in fat and sugar, and has all the necessary vitamins and minerals for good health. I love this cookbook since it gave me several alternatives and diversity for my meals, which kept me inspired and enthusiastic about my weight reduction quest. There was always a dish that suited my demands, whether I was craving something savory or sweet.

The stir-fry with turkey and vegetables was one of my favorite dishes in the cookbook. This meal was simple to prepare in about 30 minutes and was full of veggies and protein. The Greek yogurt parfait was a tasty and nutritious dessert choice that pleased my sweet desire without impeding my progress, and I really adored it. In addition to assisting me in losing weight, the Gastric Sleeve Bariatric Diet Cookbook educated me on the value of nutrition and how to make smart decisions in general. It gave me the know-how and resources I needed to develop a long-term successful sustainable and healthy lifestyle.

I heartily suggest the Gastric Sleeve Bariatric Diet Cookbook if you're considering going on a restrictive diet or have already had gastric sleeve surgery. You will have many alternatives for tasty and nutritious meals, and it will also inspire and drive you to live your best life and reach your health objectives. ----- **Claudette R. Baker**

Gastric sleeve surgery, also known as sleeve gastrectomy, is a weight reduction procedure that includes the removal of a major section of the stomach in order to lower its size and restrict the quantity of food that can be ingested. This surgical technique has grown in popularity over the years due to its effectiveness in assisting clients in achieving considerable weight reduction and improving their overall health. To optimize the effects of the treatment and prevent any negative effects, it is crucial to keep a balanced diet after having gastric sleeve surgery. In this book, we'll talk about the value of eating well following gastric sleeve surgery and provide advice on how to lead a healthy lifestyle.

Promotes Loss of Weight

After gastric sleeve surgery, weight reduction must be supported with a nutritious diet. Since the stomach is substantially smaller after the treatment, people won't be able to eat as much as they used to because they'll feel full more soon. To guarantee that the body is getting the nutrients it needs and to support long-term weight reduction, it is nonetheless crucial to consume a balanced and nutritious diet.

Decreases the likelihood of complications

After gastric sleeve surgery, maintaining a healthy diet may also assist to lower the chance of problems. For instance, eating meals heavy in fat or sugar might induce digestion problems and weight gain, which can contribute to the body's stress. These problems may be avoided, and surgical recovery can go as smoothly as possible, with the support of a balanced diet high in fruits, vegetables, lean meats, and whole grains.

Delivers Vital Nutrients

A balanced diet is crucial to provide the body the nutrition it needs to operate correctly. The body will need less calories after gastric sleeve surgery, but it will still need the same number of vitamins, minerals, and other elements to promote good health. People may make sure their body is getting the nutrients it needs to perform at its optimum by eating a balanced and nutritious diet.

Promotes General Health

After gastric sleeve surgery, maintaining a nutritious diet may help your overall health and wellbeing. A diet high in fresh produce, lean meats, and whole grains may lower your chance of developing chronic illnesses including diabetes, heart disease, and certain forms of cancer. A nutritious diet may also promote healthy digestion, lower inflammation, and increase energy levels.

Keeps Long-Term Weight Loss Up

Lastly, sustaining long-term weight reduction after gastric sleeve surgery requires sticking to a balanced diet. Although the procedure might result in rapid weight reduction in the near term, it's crucial to adjust your lifestyle and develop good habits to keep the weight off. People may reach and maintain a healthy weight for years by adhering to a nutritious diet and include regular exercise in their regimen.

Maintaining a Healthy Diet after Gastric Sleeve Surgery: Some Advice

- During the day, eat small, frequently spaced meals.
- Put an emphasis on foods high in protein, such eggs, fish, and lean meats.

- Avoid processed snacks, candies, and meals that are heavy in sugar, fat, and calories.
- To keep hydrated, drink plenty of water throughout the day.
- To make sure you are receiving enough fiber and other nutrients, include fruits and veggies in your meals.

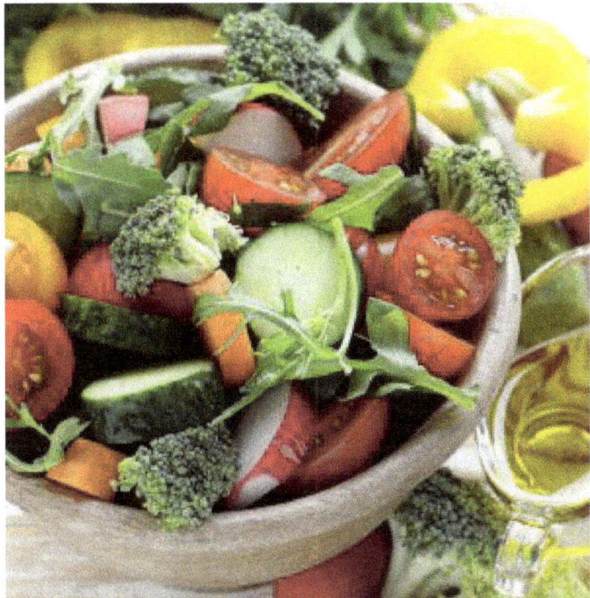

- Adopt a diet that satisfies your unique nutritional requirements.

Chapter 1: Pre-Op Diet Recipes

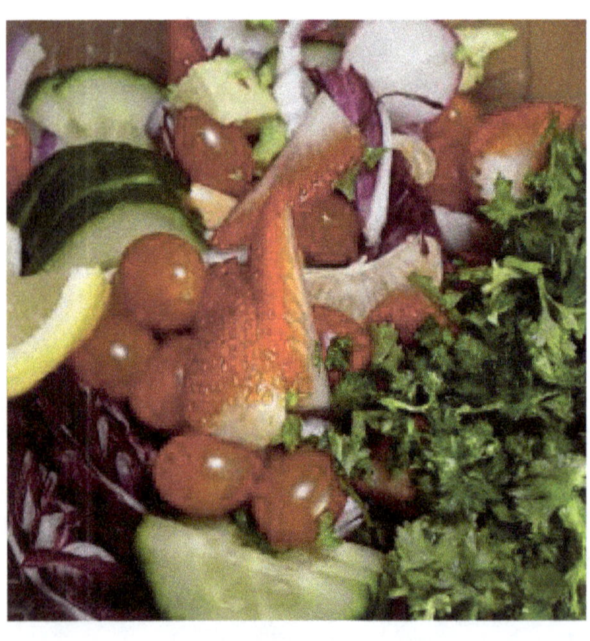

An essential part of getting ready for gastric sleeve surgery is the pre-op diet. The procedure will be safer and more successful since it will shrink your liver and lessen the amount of fat surrounding your abdomen. Pre-op diet duration might vary, but most patients adhere to it for two to four weeks before to surgery.

What does the pre-op diet include? In essence, it's a low-carb, high-protein diet. You must stay away from fried or fatty meals, as well as those high in sugar and carbohydrate. Instead, you'll consume a lot of vegetables, some fruits, and lean proteins like chicken, fish, and tofu.

Protein drinks are one of the mainstays of the pre-op diet. Usually, whey protein powder, water, or low-fat milk are used to make these drinks. They're a fantastic method to get the substantial quantities of protein you need while consuming little calories.

Hydration is a crucial component of the pre-op diet. You must consume a lot of water—at least 64 ounces daily. It also removes toxins from your body and aids in keeping you hydrated.

To receive the greatest outcomes from your operation, it's crucial to strictly adhere to the pre-op diet. It will not only help shrink your liver and decrease belly fat, but it will also assist you in creating good eating habits for after your operation.

Thus, if you're considering having a gastric sleeve, don't be put off by the pre-op diet. You may simply follow it and have your operation provide the greatest outcomes with a little planning and preparation. Moreover, for some enticing and nourishing meal suggestions, check out our Gastric Sleeve Bariatric Diet Cookbook!

PRE-OP 7 DAYS MEAL PLAN

Day 1

Breakfast:

- 1/2 cup cooked oatmeal with 1 tbsp almond butter and 1/4 cup blueberries
- 1 hard-boiled egg
- 1 cup unsweetened almond milk

Snack:

- 1 small apple
- 1 oz cheddar cheese

Lunch:

- Turkey and avocado lettuce wraps: 3 oz turkey breast, 1/2 avocado, 2 leaves of lettuce, sliced tomato, and cucumber
- 1/2 cup low-fat Greek yogurt

Snack:

- 1/4 cup hummus with 1 cup baby carrots

Dinner:

- 3 oz grilled chicken breast
- 1/2 cup cooked quinoa with 1/4 cup chopped bell pepper and 1/4 cup diced onion
- 1 cup steamed broccoli

Snack:

- 1 small pear
- 1 oz mixed nuts

Day 2

- 2 scrambled eggs with 1 oz shredded cheddar cheese
- 1/2 cup fresh berries
- 1 slice of whole grain toast

Snack:

- 1 small banana
- 1 oz almond butter

Lunch:

- Tuna salad lettuce cups: 3 oz canned tuna, 1/4 cup diced celery, 1/4 cup diced onion, 1 tbsp light mayo, 2 leaves of lettuce
- 1/2 cup low-fat cottage cheese

Snack:

- 1/4 cup roasted edamame

Dinner:

- 3 oz grilled salmon
- 1/2 cup cooked brown rice with 1/4 cup diced cucumber and 1/4 cup diced tomato
- 1 cup steamed asparagus

Snack:

- 1 small peach
- 1 oz mixed nuts

Day 3

Breakfast:

- 1/2 cup low-fat plain Greek yogurt with 1/4 cup fresh berries and 1 tbsp honey
- 1 slice of whole grain toast
- 1 cup unsweetened almond milk

Snack:

- 1 small apple
- 1 oz cheddar cheese

Lunch:

- Grilled chicken and vegetable skewers: 3 oz chicken breast, 1/4 cup sliced bell pepper, 1/4 cup sliced onion, 1/4 cup zucchini
- 1/2 cup low-fat cottage cheese

Snack:

- 1/4 cup roasted chickpeas

Dinner:

- 3 oz grilled shrimp
- 1/2 cup cooked quinoa with 1/4 cup diced cucumber and 1/4 cup diced tomato
- 1 cup steamed green beans

Snack:

- 1 small pear
- 1 oz mixed nuts

Day 4

Breakfast:

- 2 hard-boiled eggs
- 1 small orange
- 1 slice of whole grain toast

- 1 small banana
- 1 oz almond butter

Lunch:

- Turkey and cheese roll-ups: 3 oz turkey breast, 1 oz cheddar cheese, 2 leaves of lettuce
- 1/2 cup low-fat Greek yogurt

Snack:

- 1/4 cup roasted edamame

Dinner:

- 3 oz grilled chicken breast
- 1/2 cup cooked brown rice with 1/4 cup diced bell pepper and 1/4 cup diced onion
- 1 cup steamed carrots

Snack:

- 1 small apple
- 1 oz mixed nuts

Day 5

Breakfast:

- ½ cup low-fat plain Greek yogurt with 1/4 cup fresh

berries and 1 tbsp honey

- 1 hard-boiled egg
- 1 cup unsweetened almond milk

Snack:

- 1 small pear
- 1 oz cheddar cheese

Lunch:

- Chicken salad with Greek yogurt dressing: 3 oz grilled chicken breast, 1/4 cup diced cucumber, 1/4 cup diced tomato, 1 tbsp Greek yogurt dressing
- 1/2 cup low-fat cottage cheese

Snack:

- 1/4 cup hummus with 1 cup sliced cucumber

Dinner:

- 3 oz grilled salmon
- 1/2 cup cooked quinoa with 1/4 cup diced bell pepper and 1/4 cup diced onion
- 1 cup steamed broccoli

Snack:

- 1 small banana
- 1 oz mixed nuts

Day 6

Breakfast:

- 2 scrambled eggs with 1 oz shredded cheddar cheese
- 1/2 cup fresh berries

- 1 slice of whole grain toast

- 1 small apple
- 1 oz almond butter

Lunch:

- Grilled chicken and vegetable skewers: 3 oz chicken breast, 1/4 cup sliced bell pepper, 1/4 cup sliced onion, 1/4 cup zucchini
- 1/2 cup low-fat Greek yogurt

Snack:

- 1/4 cup roasted chickpeas

Dinner:

- 3 oz grilled shrimp
- 1/2 cup cooked brown rice with 1/4 cup diced cucumber and 1/4 cup diced tomato
- 1 cup steamed green beans

Snack:

- 1 small pear
- 1 oz mixed nuts

Day 7

Breakfast:

- 1/2 cup cooked oatmeal with 1 tbsp almond butter and 1/4 cup blueberries
- 1 hard-boiled egg
- 1 cup unsweetened almond milk

Snack:

- 1 small apple
- 1 oz cheddar cheese

Lunch:

- Turkey and avocado lettuce wraps: 3 oz turkey breast, 1/2 avocado, 2 leaves of lettuce, sliced tomato, and cucumber
- 1/2 cup low-fat Greek yogurt

Snack:

- 1/4 cup hummus with 1 cup baby carrots

Dinner:

- 3 oz grilled chicken breast
- 1/2 cup cooked quinoa with 1/4 cup chopped bell pepper and 1/4 cup diced onion
- 1 cup steamed broccoli

Snack:

- 1 small peach
- 1 oz mixed nuts

PRE-OP BREAKFAST RECIPES

SCRAMBLED EGGS WITH SPINACH AND FETA

Ingredients:

- 2 large eggs
- 1/4 cup fresh spinach, chopped
- 1 tbsp crumbled feta cheese
- Salt and pepper to taste
- Cooking spray

Cooking Guidelines :

1) In a small mixing bowl, whisk the eggs until the yolks and whites are combined.
2) Add the chopped spinach and crumbled feta cheese to the bowl, and mix well with the eggs.
3) Heat a non-stick skillet over medium heat and spray with cooking spray.
4) Pour the egg mixture into the skillet and let it cook for a minute or two.
5) Use a spatula to scramble the eggs until they are cooked through.
6) Sprinkle with salt and pepper to taste.
7) Serve with a small portion size of approximately 1/2 to 3/4 cup per serving.

GREEK YOGURT WITH FRESH BERRIES AND ALMONDS

Ingredients:

- 1/2 cup plain nonfat Greek yogurt
- 1/2 cup fresh berries (such as strawberries, blueberries, or raspberries)
- 1 tbsp slivered almonds
- 1 tsp honey (optional)

Cooking Guidelines :

1) In a small bowl, add the Greek yogurt.
2) Wash the fresh berries and add them to the bowl.
3) Sprinkle the slivered almonds over the top of the berries and yogurt.
4) If desired, drizzle honey over the top.
5) Serve with a small portion size of approximately ½ cup per serving.

OATMEAL WITH CHIA SEEDS AND BANANA

Ingredients:

- 1/2 cup rolled oats
- 1 cup water
- 1 tbsp chia seeds
- 1 small banana, sliced
- Cinnamon to taste
- 1 tsp honey (optional)

Cooking Guidelines :

1) In a small saucepan, add the rolled oats and water and bring to a boil.
2) Reduce heat and let the oats simmer for 5-10 minutes, stirring occasionally, until they reach your desired consistency.
3) Remove from heat and stir in the chia seeds.
4) Add the sliced banana to the top of the oatmeal.
5) Sprinkle cinnamon over the top of the banana and oatmeal.
6) If desired, drizzle honey over the top.

7) Serve with a small portion size of approximately ½ cup per serving.

BREAKFAST TACOS WITH TURKEY SAUSAGE AND AVOCADO

Ingredients:

- 2 small whole wheat tortillas
- 2 turkey sausage patties, cooked and crumbled
- 2 eggs, scrambled
- 1/4 avocado, sliced
- Salsa (optional)
- Salt and pepper to taste

Cooking Guidelines :

1) Heat the tortillas in a dry skillet or in the microwave for 10-15 seconds to warm them up.
2) Cook the turkey sausage patties according to the package Cooking Guidelines , then crumble them into small pieces.
3) In a small bowl, whisk the eggs and scramble them in a non-stick skillet over medium heat.
4) To assemble the tacos, divide the scrambled eggs and crumbled turkey sausage evenly between the two tortillas.
5) Top each taco with sliced avocado.
6) Add a spoonful of salsa, if desired.

7) Sprinkle salt and pepper over the top of the tacos.
8) Serve with a portion size of approximately 1 taco per serving.

COTTAGE CHEESE WITH PINEAPPLE AND WALNUTS

Ingredients:

- 1/2 cup low-fat cottage cheese
- 1/2 cup fresh pineapple chunks
- 1 tbsp chopped walnuts
- Cinnamon to taste

Cooking Guidelines :

1) In a small mixing bowl, add the cottage cheese.
2) Add the fresh pineapple chunks to the bowl and mix well.
3) Sprinkle the chopped walnuts over the top of the cottage cheese and pineapple mixture.
4) Sprinkle cinnamon over the top of the mixture.
5) Serve with a portion size of approximately 1/2 cup per serving.

PROTEIN SHAKE WITH SPINACH AND PEANUT BUTTER

Ingredients:

- 1 scoop vanilla protein powder
- 1 cup unsweetened almond milk
- 1/2 banana
- 1 tbsp natural peanut butter
- 1 cup fresh spinach leaves
- Ice cubes (optional)

Cooking Guidelines :

1) In a blender, add the vanilla protein powder and unsweetened almond milk.
2) Add the banana, natural peanut butter, and fresh spinach leaves.
3) If desired, add a few ice cubes to the blender to make the shake colder.
4) Blend all the ingredients together until smooth.
5) Pour the protein shake into a glass and serve with a portion size of approximately 1 cup per serving.

BROILED GRAPEFRUIT WITH CINNAMON AND HONEY

Ingredients:

- 1 large grapefruit, halved
- 1/2 tsp cinnamon
- 1 tbsp honey

Cooking Guidelines :

1) Preheat the oven to broil.
2) Cut the grapefruit in half and use a small knife to cut around the edges of the fruit to loosen it from the

skin.

3) Sprinkle cinnamon over the top of each grapefruit
half.

4) Drizzle honey over the top of the grapefruit halves.

5) Place the grapefruit halves on a baking sheet and broil
in the oven for 3-5 minutes, or until the top is lightly
browned and bubbly.

6) Remove the grapefruit from the oven and let it cool
for a minute or two.

7) Serve the broiled grapefruit with a portion size of one
half grapefruit per serving.

SWEET POTATO HASH WITH TURKEY BACON AND EGGS

Ingredients:

- 1 large sweet potato, peeled and diced
- 2 slices turkey bacon, chopped
- 2 eggs
- 1/2 small onion, chopped
- 1/2 red bell pepper, chopped
- Salt and pepper to taste
- 1 tbsp olive oil

Cooking Guidelines :

1) Heat a non-stick skillet over medium heat and add the
olive oil.

2) Add the chopped onion and red bell pepper to the
skillet and cook until softened.

3) Add the chopped turkey bacon to the skillet and cook
until crispy.

4) Add the diced sweet potato to the skillet and cook until tender and lightly browned.
5) In a separate pan, fry the eggs until the yolks are cooked to your preference.
6) To serve, divide the sweet potato hash evenly between two plates.
7) Top each plate with a fried egg.
8) Sprinkle salt and pepper over the top of the eggs.
9) Serve with a portion size of approximately 1 cup of sweet potato hash and 1 egg per serving.

QUINOA BREAKFAST BOWL WITH ALMOND BUTTER AND FRUIT

Ingredients:

- 1/2 cup cooked quinoa
- 1 tbsp almond butter
- 1/2 banana, sliced
- 1/2 cup mixed berries (such as strawberries, blueberries, and raspberries)
- 1 tbsp chopped almonds
- 1 tsp honey (optional)

Cooking Guidelines :

1) In a bowl, add the cooked quinoa.
2) Add the almond butter to the bowl and mix well.
3) Add the sliced banana and mixed berries to the bowl.
4) Sprinkle chopped almonds over the top of the quinoa bowl.
5) If desired, drizzle honey over the top of the quinoa bowl for added sweetness.

6) Serve with a portion size of approximately 1 cup per
   serving.

TURKEY SAUSAGE AND EGG MUFFINS

Ingredients:

- 4 large eggs
- 1/4 cup unsweetened almond milk
- 1/2 cup cooked and crumbled turkey sausage
- 1/4 cup shredded cheddar cheese
- Salt and pepper to taste
- Cooking spray

Cooking Guidelines :

1) Preheat the oven to 375°F.
2) In a mixing bowl, beat the eggs and almond milk
   together until well combined.
3) Add the cooked turkey sausage and shredded cheddar
   cheese to the bowl.
4) Mix the ingredients together until they are evenly
   distributed.
5) Season the mixture with salt and pepper to taste.
6) Spray a muffin tin with cooking spray.
7) Pour the egg mixture into the muffin cups, filling each
   cup about 2/3 full.
8) Bake the muffins in the oven for 20-25 minutes, or
   until the eggs are cooked through and the tops are
   lightly browned.
9) Remove the muffins from the oven and let them cool
   for a few minutes.
10) Use a knife or spatula to loosen the muffins from the

tin and remove them from the pan.

11) Serve with a portion size of 2 muffins per serving.

Pre-op Lunch Recipes

CHICKEN CAESAR SALAD

Ingredients:

- 4 oz boneless, skinless chicken breast
- 1/2 head of romaine lettuce, chopped
- 1/4 cup of freshly grated parmesan cheese
- 1/4 cup of low-fat Caesar dressing
- 1/4 cup of croutons (optional)

Cooking Guidelines :

1) Preheat the oven to 375°F.
2) Season the chicken breast with salt and pepper and place it on a baking sheet lined with parchment paper.
3) Bake the chicken breast in the oven for 20-25 minutes or until the internal temperature reaches 165°F.
4) Remove the chicken breast from the oven and let it cool for 5-10 minutes.
5) Cut the chicken breast into small pieces or strips.
6) In a large bowl, add the chopped romaine lettuce and the chicken breast.
7) Add the freshly grated parmesan cheese to the bowl.
8) Add the low-fat Caesar dressing to the bowl and mix all ingredients until the salad is well coated.
9) Top the salad with croutons if desired.

TUNA SALAD LETTUCE WRAPS

Ingredients:

- 1 can of tuna in water, drained
- 1/4 cup of finely chopped celery
- 1/4 cup of finely chopped onion
- 1 tablespoon of low-fat mayonnaise
- 1 tablespoon of Dijon mustard
- Salt and pepper, to taste
- 4 large lettuce leaves (such as romaine or iceberg)

Cooking Guidelines :

1) In a small bowl, mix together the drained tuna, chopped celery, chopped onion, low-fat mayonnaise, Dijon mustard, salt, and pepper until well combined.
2) Lay the lettuce leaves flat on a plate.
3) Divide the tuna salad evenly among the four lettuce leaves.
4) Wrap each lettuce leaf around the tuna salad, folding the sides in like a burrito.
5) Serve.

TURKEY AND CHEESE ROLL-UPS

Ingredients:

- 2 oz. sliced turkey breast
- 1 oz. low-fat cheese, sliced

- 2 leaves of lettuce
- 1 tsp. mustard
- Salt and pepper to taste

Cooking Guidelines :

1) Lay out two lettuce leaves on a cutting board.
2) Spread 1/2 tsp. of mustard on each lettuce leaf.
3) Place 1 oz. of sliced cheese on each lettuce leaf.
4) Top each lettuce leaf with 1 oz. of sliced turkey breast.
5) Season with salt and pepper to taste.
6) Roll up the lettuce leaves tightly around the turkey and cheese filling.
7) Use a toothpick to secure the roll-ups.
8) Cut each roll-up in half.
9) Serve

CAULIFLOWER FRIED RICE WITH SHRIMP

Ingredients:

- 1/2 lb. shrimp, peeled and deveined
- 2 cups cauliflower rice
- 1/2 cup diced onion
- 1/2 cup diced carrot
- 1/2 cup frozen peas
- 1 clove garlic, minced
- 1 tbsp. low-sodium soy sauce
- 1 tsp. sesame oil
- 1 tsp. olive oil
- Salt and pepper to taste

Cooking Guidelines :

1) In a large skillet, heat 1 tsp. of olive oil over medium-high heat.
2) Add the shrimp to the skillet and cook for 2-3 minutes on each side until pink and cooked through. Remove the shrimp from the skillet and set aside.
3) In the same skillet, add the diced onion and carrot. Cook for 3-4 minutes until tender.
4) Add the minced garlic and cook for an additional minute.
5) Add the frozen peas to the skillet and cook for 2-3 minutes until heated through.
6) Add the cauliflower rice to the skillet and stir to combine.
7) Add the cooked shrimp back to the skillet and stir to combine.
8) Drizzle 1 tsp. of sesame oil and 1 tbsp. of low-sodium soy sauce over the skillet and stir to coat.
9) Season with salt and pepper to taste.
10) Cook for an additional 2-3 minutes until heated through.
11) Serve

LENTIL SOUP WITH SPINACH AND CARROTS

Ingredients:

- 1 cup dried lentils, rinsed and drained
- 4 cups low-sodium chicken or vegetable broth
- 1 cup diced onion
- 1 cup diced carrot
- 2 cups fresh spinach, washed and chopped
- 1 clove garlic, minced

- 1 tsp. olive oil
- Salt and pepper to taste

Cooking Guidelines :

1) In a large pot, heat 1 tsp. of olive oil over medium-high heat.
2) Add the diced onion and carrot to the pot. Cook for 3-4 minutes until tender.
3) Add the minced garlic and cook for an additional minute.
4) Add the rinsed and drained lentils to the pot.
5) Pour in the low-sodium chicken or vegetable broth and bring the mixture to a boil.
6) Reduce the heat to low and let the soup simmer for 25-30 minutes, or until the lentils are tender.
7) Stir in the chopped spinach and cook for an additional 2-3 minutes until wilted.
8) Season with salt and pepper to taste.
9) Serve

GRILLED CHICKEN AND VEGGIE SKEWERS

Ingredients:

- 1 lb. boneless, skinless chicken breasts, cut into bite-sized pieces
- 1 large zucchini, cut into bite-sized pieces
- 1 large red bell pepper, cut into bite-sized pieces
- 1 large yellow bell pepper, cut into bite-sized pieces
- 1 small red onion, cut into bite-sized pieces
- 1 tbsp. olive oil

- 1 tsp. dried oregano
- 1/2 tsp. garlic powder
- Salt and pepper to taste

Cooking Guidelines :

1) Preheat the grill to medium-high heat.
2) Thread the chicken, zucchini, red bell pepper, yellow bell pepper, and red onion onto skewers.
3) In a small bowl, whisk together the olive oil, dried oregano, garlic powder, salt, and pepper.
4) Brush the skewers with the olive oil mixture.
5) Place the skewers on the grill and cook for 10-12 minutes, turning occasionally, until the chicken is cooked through and the vegetables are tender.
6) Serve

QUINOA AND BLACK BEAN SALAD

Ingredients:

- 1 cup cooked quinoa
- 1 can black beans, rinsed and drained
- 1 large tomato, diced
- 1 small red onion, diced
- 1/4 cup chopped fresh cilantro
- 1 tbsp. olive oil
- 1 tbsp. fresh lime juice
- 1/2 tsp. ground cumin
- Salt and pepper to taste

Cooking Guidelines :

1) In a large bowl, combine the cooked quinoa, black beans, tomato, red onion, and cilantro.
2) In a small bowl, whisk together the olive oil, lime juice, ground cumin, salt, and pepper.
3) Pour the dressing over the quinoa and black bean mixture and toss to combine.
4) Serve

CUCUMBER AND AVOCADO SOUP

Ingredients:

- 2 large cucumbers, peeled and seeded
- 1 large avocado, peeled and pitted
- 1 cup low-sodium chicken or vegetable broth
- 1/4 cup chopped fresh cilantro
- 2 tbsp. fresh lime juice
- 1 clove garlic, minced
- Salt and pepper to taste

Cooking Guidelines :

1) In a blender or food processor, combine the peeled and seeded cucumbers, avocado, low-sodium chicken or vegetable broth, chopped cilantro, fresh lime juice, minced garlic, salt, and pepper.
2) Blend the mixture until smooth and creamy.
3) Pour the soup into a large bowl and chill in the refrigerator for at least 30 minutes.
4) Serve

TURKEY CHILI WITH SWEET POTATO

Ingredients:

- 1 lb. ground turkey
- 1 large sweet potato, peeled and diced
- 1 can diced tomatoes
- 1 can low-sodium black beans, rinsed and drained
- 1 small red onion, diced
- 1 green bell pepper, diced
- 1 tbsp. olive oil
- 1 tsp. chili powder
- 1/2 tsp. ground cumin
- 1/2 tsp. smoked paprika
- Salt and pepper to taste

Cooking Guidelines :

1) In a large pot, heat the olive oil over medium heat.
2) Add the ground turkey, chili powder, ground cumin, smoked paprika, salt, and pepper. Cook the turkey, stirring occasionally, until browned and cooked through.
3) Add the diced sweet potato, diced tomatoes, low-sodium black beans, diced red onion, and diced green bell pepper to the pot.
4) Bring the mixture to a simmer and cook for 20-25 minutes, stirring occasionally, until the sweet potato is tender and the flavors have melded together.
5) Serve

EGG SALAD LETTUCE WRAPS

Ingredients:

- 4 large eggs, hard-boiled and peeled
- 2 tbsp. plain Greek yogurt
- 1 tbsp. Dijon mustard
- 1 stalk celery, finely diced
- 1 small red onion, finely diced
- 2 tbsp. chopped fresh parsley
- Salt and pepper to taste
- Lettuce leaves for wrapping

Cooking Guidelines :

1) In a medium bowl, mash the hard-boiled eggs with a fork until they are crumbled into small pieces.
2) Add the plain Greek yogurt, Dijon mustard, finely diced celery, finely diced red onion, chopped fresh parsley, salt, and pepper to the bowl. Mix well to combine.
3) Place a lettuce leaf on a plate and spoon the egg salad mixture onto the center of the lettuce leaf.
4) Wrap the lettuce leaf around the egg salad mixture, folding the sides in and rolling it up.
5) Serve

EDAMAME SALAD

Ingredients:

- 2 cups cooked and shelled edamame
- 1/2 cup diced red bell pepper

- 1/2 cup diced yellow bell pepper
- 1/4 cup diced red onion
- 1/4 cup chopped fresh cilantro
- 2 tablespoons extra-virgin olive oil
- 2 tablespoons rice vinegar
- 1 tablespoon honey
- Salt and pepper to taste

Cooking Guidelines :

1) In a large mixing bowl, combine cooked edamame, red and yellow bell peppers, red onion, and cilantro.
2) In a separate small mixing bowl, whisk together olive oil, rice vinegar, honey, salt, and pepper.
3) Pour the dressing over the edamame mixture and toss to coat evenly.

Pre-op Dinner Recipes

GRILLED CHICKEN BREAST WITH ROASTED VEGETABLES

Ingredients:

- 2 skinless, boneless chicken breasts
- 2 cups mixed vegetables (such as bell peppers, zucchini, and onion), cut into bite-sized pieces
- 1 tbsp. olive oil
- 1 tsp. garlic powder
- 1 tsp. dried oregano
- Salt and pepper to taste

Cooking Guidelines :

1) Preheat the oven to 400°F (200°C).
2) Place the chicken breasts on a plate and season both sides with garlic powder, dried oregano, salt, and pepper.
3) In a separate bowl, toss the mixed vegetables with the olive oil and a pinch of salt and pepper.
4) Grill the chicken breasts on a preheated grill or grill pan for 4-5 minutes per side, or until they are cooked through.
5) Place the vegetables on a baking sheet and roast in the preheated oven for 15-20 minutes, or until they are tender and slightly browned.
6) Serve the grilled chicken breasts with the roasted vegetables on the side.

BAKED SALMON WITH BROCCOLI AND QUINOA

Ingredients:

- 4 oz salmon fillet
- 1 cup broccoli florets
- 1/4 cup uncooked quinoa
- 1/2 cup low-sodium chicken broth
- 1/4 teaspoon salt
- 1/4 teaspoon black pepper
- 1/4 teaspoon garlic powder
- 1/4 teaspoon paprika
- 1 tablespoon olive oil

Cooking Guidelines :

1) Preheat the oven to 375°F.
2) Rinse the quinoa and add it to a small saucepan with the chicken broth and a pinch of salt. Bring to a boil, then reduce the heat to low and simmer for 15 minutes, or until the liquid is absorbed and the quinoa is cooked through.
3) While the quinoa is cooking, steam the broccoli for 5-7 minutes, or until tender but still firm.
4) Season the salmon fillet with the salt, black pepper, garlic powder, and paprika.
5) Heat the olive oil in a large oven-safe skillet over medium-high heat. When the oil is hot, add the salmon fillet to the skillet, skin side down. Cook for 3-4 minutes, or until the skin is crispy.
6) Flip the salmon fillet over and transfer the skillet to the preheated oven. Bake for 10-12 minutes, or until the salmon is cooked through.
7) Serve the baked salmon with the steamed broccoli and quinoa.

TACO-STUFFED PEPPERS

Ingredients:

- 2 large bell peppers, halved and seeded
- 1/2 pound lean ground turkey
- 1/2 cup diced onion
- 1/2 cup diced tomato
- 1/2 cup canned black beans, drained and rinsed
- 1/2 cup cooked brown rice
- 1/2 teaspoon chili powder
- 1/2 teaspoon cumin

- 1/4 teaspoon garlic powder
- 1/4 teaspoon onion powder
- Salt and pepper, to taste
- 1/4 cup shredded cheddar cheese
- 1 tablespoon chopped fresh cilantro

Cooking Guidelines :

1) Preheat the oven to 375°F.
2) Place the pepper halves cut side up in a baking dish and bake for 15 minutes.
3) While the peppers are baking, cook the ground turkey and onion in a large skillet over medium-high heat until the turkey is browned and the onion is tender, about 5-7 minutes.
4) Add the tomato, black beans, brown rice, chili powder, cumin, garlic powder, onion powder, salt, and pepper to the skillet with the turkey and onion. Stir well to combine and heat through.
5) When the peppers are done baking, remove them from the oven and spoon the turkey mixture into each pepper half, filling them as much as possible.
6) Top each pepper half with a sprinkle of shredded cheddar cheese.
7) Return the peppers to the oven and bake for an additional 10-15 minutes, or until the cheese is melted and the peppers are tender.
8) Garnish with chopped fresh cilantro and divide into appropriate portions (such as one pepper half per serving).

SHRIMP STIR-FRY WITH BROWN RICE

Ingredients:

- 1/2 cup uncooked brown rice
- 1 cup low-sodium chicken broth
- 1 tablespoon olive oil
- 1/2 pound shrimp, peeled and deveined
- 1 cup sliced mushrooms
- 1 cup sliced bell pepper
- 1/2 cup sliced onion
- 1/2 cup sliced carrots
- 1/2 cup chopped broccoli florets
- 1/2 teaspoon garlic powder
- Salt and pepper, to taste
- 1 tablespoon low-sodium soy sauce
- 1 tablespoon chopped fresh cilantro

Cooking Guidelines :

1) Rinse the brown rice and add it to a small saucepan with the chicken broth and a pinch of salt. Bring to a boil, then reduce the heat to low and simmer for 40-45 minutes, or until the liquid is absorbed and the rice is cooked through.
2) While the rice is cooking, heat the olive oil in a large skillet or wok over high heat. Add the shrimp and stir-fry for 2-3 minutes, or until pink and cooked through. Remove the shrimp from the skillet and set aside.
3) Add the mushrooms, bell pepper, onion, carrots, and broccoli to the skillet and stir-fry for 4-5 minutes, or until the vegetables are tender-crisp.
4) Season the vegetables with the garlic powder, salt, and pepper, then add the cooked shrimp back to the skillet.
5) Drizzle the low-sodium soy sauce over the stir-fry and

stir well to combine.

6) Serve the shrimp stir-fry over the cooked brown rice,
   Garnish with chopped fresh cilantro.

ZUCCHINI NOODLE PASTA WITH TURKEY MEATBALLS

Ingredients:

- 2 medium zucchinis, spiraled or cut into thin strips
- 1/2 pound lean ground turkey
- 1/4 cup almond flour
- 1 egg
- 1/2 teaspoon garlic powder
- 1/2 teaspoon dried oregano
- Salt and pepper, to taste
- 1 tablespoon olive oil
- 1 cup low-sodium tomato sauce
- 1/4 cup grated parmesan cheese
- Chopped fresh parsley, for garnish

Cooking Guidelines :

1) Preheat the oven to 400°F.
2) In a large mixing bowl, combine the ground turkey,
   almond flour, egg, garlic powder, dried oregano, salt,
   and pepper. Mix well to combine.
3) Form the turkey mixture into small meatballs, about 1
   inch in diameter.
4) Heat the olive oil in a large skillet over medium-high
   heat. Add the meatballs to the skillet and cook for 3-4
   minutes, or until browned on all sides.

5) Transfer the meatballs to a baking dish and bake in the preheated oven for 10-15 minutes, or until cooked through.

6) While the meatballs are baking, add the zucchini noodles to the skillet and sauté over medium heat for 2-3 minutes, or until tender.

7) Add the tomato sauce to the skillet with the zucchini noodles and stir well to combine. Heat through.

8) To serve, divide the zucchini noodle mixture onto plates or bowls, top with the turkey meatballs, and sprinkle with grated parmesan cheese and chopped fresh parsley.

BLACKENED TILAPIA WITH CABBAGE SLAW

Ingredients:

- 4 tilapia fillets
- 2 teaspoons paprika
- 1 teaspoon garlic powder
- 1/2 teaspoon onion powder
- 1/2 teaspoon dried thyme
- 1/2 teaspoon dried oregano
- 1/4 teaspoon cayenne pepper
- Salt and pepper, to taste
- 1 tablespoon olive oil
- 1/2 small head of cabbage, thinly sliced
- 1/2 red onion, thinly sliced
- 1/2 red bell pepper, thinly sliced
- 2 tablespoons apple cider vinegar
- 1 tablespoon honey

- 1 tablespoon Dijon mustard
- 1 tablespoon olive oil
- Salt and pepper, to taste

Cooking Guidelines :

1) Preheat the oven to 400°F.
2) In a small bowl, mix together the paprika, garlic powder, onion powder, dried thyme, dried oregano, cayenne pepper, salt, and pepper.
3) Rub the tilapia fillets with the spice mixture, coating both sides.
4) Heat the olive oil in a large oven-safe skillet over high heat. Add the tilapia fillets and cook for 2-3 minutes per side, or until blackened.
5) Transfer the skillet to the preheated oven and bake for 5-7 minutes, or until the tilapia is cooked through.
6) While the tilapia is cooking, make the cabbage slaw. In a large mixing bowl, combine the sliced cabbage, red onion, and red bell pepper.
7) In a small bowl, whisk together the apple cider vinegar, honey, Dijon mustard, olive oil, salt, and pepper.
8) Pour the dressing over the cabbage mixture and toss well to combine.
9) Serve the blackened tilapia with the cabbage slaw on the side.

CHICKEN AND VEGETABLE SKILLET

Ingredients:

- 2 boneless, skinless chicken breasts, cut into bite-sized pieces

- 1 tablespoon olive oil
- 1/2 small onion, diced
- 1 red bell pepper, sliced
- 1 zucchini, slice.
- 1 yellow squash, sliced
- 2 cloves garlic, minced
- Salt and pepper, to taste
- 1/2 teaspoon dried thyme
- 1/2 teaspoon dried rosemary
- 1/4 teaspoon paprika
- 1/4 cup low-sodium chicken broth

Cooking Guidelines :

1) Heat the olive oil in a large skillet over medium-high heat. Add the chicken and cook for 5-7 minutes, or until browned on all sides.
2) Add the onion, red bell pepper, zucchini, and yellow squash to the skillet with the chicken. Cook for 5-7 minutes, or until the vegetables are tender.
3) Add the garlic to the skillet and cook for an additional 1-2 minutes, or until fragrant.
4) Season the chicken and vegetables with salt, pepper, dried thyme, dried rosemary, and paprika. Stir well to combine.
5) Pour the chicken broth into the skillet and stir well. Bring to a simmer and cook for 2-3 minutes, or until the liquid has reduced slightly.
6) Serve the chicken and vegetable skillet hot.

GRILLED STEAK WITH ASPARAGUS

Ingredients:

- 2 beef tenderloin steaks, about 4-5 oz each
- Salt and pepper, to taste
- 1 tablespoon olive oil
- 1 bunch asparagus, trimmed
- 1 tablespoon balsamic vinegar
- 1 tablespoon Dijon mustard
- 1 tablespoon olive oil
- Salt and pepper, to taste

Cooking Guidelines :

1) Preheat the grill to high heat.
2) Season the steaks with salt and pepper, and brush them with olive oil.
3) Grill the steaks for 3-4 minutes per side, or until cooked to your desired level of doneness.
4) While the steaks are cooking, prepare the asparagus. In a small bowl, whisk together the balsamic vinegar, Dijon mustard, olive oil, salt, and pepper.
5) Place the asparagus on the grill and brush with the balsamic mixture. Grill for 2-3 minutes per side, or until tender.
6) Serve the grilled steak with the grilled asparagus on the side.

STUFFED PORTOBELLO MUSHROOM CAPS

Ingredients:

- 4 large portobello mushroom caps
- 1 tablespoon olive oil

- 1/2 small onion, diced
- 1 red bell pepper, diced
- 2 cloves garlic, minced
- 1/2 teaspoon dried oregano
- 1/2 teaspoon dried thyme
- 1/2 teaspoon paprika
- Salt and pepper, to taste
- 1/4 cup low-sodium chicken broth
- 4 oz ground turkey
- 1/4 cup grated parmesan cheese

Cooking Guidelines :

1) Preheat the oven to 375°F.
2) Clean the portobello mushroom caps and remove the stems. Set them aside.
3) In a large skillet, heat the olive oil over medium-high heat. Add the onion, red bell pepper, and garlic to the skillet and cook for 2-3 minutes, or until the vegetables are tender.
4) Add the ground turkey to the skillet and cook until browned, stirring occasionally.
5) Add the dried oregano, dried thyme, paprika, salt, and pepper to the skillet. Stir well to combine.
6) Pour the chicken broth into the skillet and stir well. Bring to a simmer and cook for 2-3 minutes, or until the liquid has reduced slightly.
7) Place the portobello mushroom caps on a baking sheet lined with parchment paper. Spoon the turkey and vegetable mixture into the mushroom caps.
8) Sprinkle the grated parmesan cheese over the top of the stuffed mushroom caps.
9) Bake the stuffed mushroom caps in the preheated oven for 15-20 minutes, or until the mushrooms are

tender and the cheese is melted and bubbly.
10) Serve the stuffed portobello mushroom caps hot.

TURKEY BURGER WITH SWEET POTATO FRIES

Ingredients:

For the turkey burger:

- 4 oz ground turkey breast
- Salt and pepper, to taste
- 1 tablespoon olive oil
- 1 small onion, sliced
- 1/2 avocado, sliced
- 2 small whole wheat buns or lettuce wraps

For the sweet potato fries:

- 1 medium sweet potato, cut into thin fries
- 1 tablespoon olive oil
- Salt and pepper, to taste

Cooking Guidelines :

1) Preheat the oven to 425°F.
2) In a bowl, season the ground turkey breast with salt and pepper, then shape it into two patties.
3) Heat the olive oil in a nonstick pan over medium-high heat, then add the patties and cook for 3-4 minutes on each side or until fully cooked.
4) Meanwhile, prepare the sweet potato fries by spreading them in a single layer on a baking sheet lined with parchment paper.
5) Drizzle the sweet potato fries with olive oil, then

sprinkle with salt and pepper.

6) Roast the sweet potato fries in the preheated oven for 15-20 minutes, or until they are tender and crispy.
7) Assemble the turkey burger by placing the cooked patty on a whole wheat bun or lettuce wrap, and adding sliced onion and avocado.
8) Serve the turkey burger with the sweet potato fries on the side.

Pre-op Snack Recipes

APPLE SLICES WITH ALMOND BUTTER

Ingredients:

- 1 medium apple
- 1 tablespoon almond butter

Cooking Guidelines :

1) Wash the apple and cut it into thin slices.
2) Spread the almond butter evenly over the apple slices.

GREEK YOGURT WITH BERRIES

Ingredients:

- 1/2 cup of plain Greek yogurt
- 1/2 cup of mixed berries (such as strawberries, blueberries, raspberries)

- 1 tablespoon of honey (optional)

Cooking Guidelines :

1) Rinse the berries and chop any larger ones into bite-sized pieces.
2) In a small bowl, mix the Greek yogurt with honey (if using) until well combined.
3) Add the mixed berries on top of the yogurt mixture.
4) Serve.

STRING CHEESE WITH CHERRY TOMATOES

Ingredients:

- 2 string cheese sticks
- 1 cup cherry tomatoes, halved
- 1 tbsp balsamic vinegar
- 1 tbsp extra-virgin olive oil
- Salt and pepper, to taste
- Fresh basil leaves, for garnish

Cooking Guidelines :

1) Cut the string cheese sticks into bite-sized pieces.
2) In a small bowl, whisk together the balsamic vinegar, olive oil, salt, and pepper.
3) In a separate bowl, mix the cherry tomato halves with the balsamic vinaigrette.
4) Thread the cheese pieces and cherry tomatoes onto skewers or toothpicks, alternating them.
5) Garnish with fresh basil leaves before serving.

HUMMUS AND CARROT STICKS

Ingredients:

- 1 can of chickpeas, drained and rinsed
- 2 garlic cloves, minced
- 2 tbsp tahini
- 2 tbsp lemon juice
- 2 tbsp extra-virgin olive oil
- Salt and pepper, to taste
- 1/2 tsp ground cumin
- Carrot sticks, for serving

Cooking Guidelines :

1) In a food processor or blender, combine the chickpeas, garlic, tahini, lemon juice, olive oil, salt, pepper, and cumin. Blend until smooth.
2) If the mixture is too thick, add a little bit of water until it reaches your desired consistency.
3) Serve the hummus with the carrot sticks.

HARD-BOILED EGG

Ingredients:

- 2 large eggs
- Salt and pepper, to taste

Cooking Guidelines :

1) Place the eggs in a saucepan and cover them with cold water. The water should be about 1 inch above the

eggs.
2) Bring the water to a boil over high heat.
3) Once the water is boiling, remove the saucepan from the heat and cover it with a lid.
4) Let the eggs sit in the hot water for about 9-12 minutes, depending on how you like your yolks.
5) After the time has elapsed, remove the eggs from the hot water and place them in a bowl of cold water to cool for a few minutes.
6) Peel the eggs and season them with salt and pepper to taste.

COTTAGE CHEESE WITH PINEAPPLE

Ingredients:

- 1/2 cup low-fat cottage cheese
- 1/2 cup fresh pineapple chunks
- 1 tbsp honey
- 1/4 tsp vanilla extract

Cooking Guidelines :

1) In a small bowl, mix together the cottage cheese, honey, and vanilla extract.
2) Add the fresh pineapple chunks on top of the cottage cheese mixture.
3) Serve chilled.

TURKEY JERKY

Ingredients:

- 8 large lettuce leaves
- 1/2 pound turkey jerky, shredded
- 1/2 cup shredded carrots
- 1/2 cup diced cucumber
- 1/4 cup diced red onion
- 1/4 cup chopped fresh cilantro
- 2 tablespoons low-sodium soy sauce
- 2 tablespoons rice vinegar
- 1 tablespoon honey
- 1 tablespoon sesame oil

Cooking Guidelines :

1) In a large mixing bowl, combine shredded turkey jerky, shredded carrots, diced cucumber, red onion, and cilantro.
2) In a separate small mixing bowl, whisk together soy sauce, rice vinegar, honey, and sesame oil.
3) Pour the dressing over the turkey jerky mixture and toss to coat evenly.
4) Spoon the turkey jerky mixture onto the lettuce leaves and wrap the lettuce leaves around the filling to make lettuce wraps.
5) Serve

ROASTED CHICKPEAS

Ingredients:

- 2 cups cooked chickpeas
- 1 cup cherry tomatoes, halved

- 1/2 cup diced cucumber
- 1/4 cup diced red onion
- 1/4 cup chopped fresh parsley
- 2 tablespoons extra-virgin olive oil
- 2 tablespoons lemon juice
- 1 teaspoon ground cumin
- Salt and pepper to taste

Cooking Guidelines :

1) Preheat the oven to 400°F.
2) Drain and rinse the cooked chickpeas and pat them dry with a paper towel. Spread the chickpeas out on a baking sheet and drizzle with 1 tablespoon of olive oil. Season with cumin, salt, and pepper to taste.
3) Roast the chickpeas in the oven for 20-25 minutes, or until they are crispy and lightly browned.
4) In a large mixing bowl, combine the roasted chickpeas, cherry tomatoes, diced cucumber, red onion, and parsley.
5) In a separate small mixing bowl, whisk together the remaining tablespoon of olive oil and lemon juice.
6) Pour the dressing over the chickpea mixture and toss to coat evenly.
7) Serve.

BEEF JERKY WITH ALMONDS

Ingredients:

- 1 pound lean beef (such as flank steak)
- 1/4 cup low-sodium soy sauce

- 2 tablespoons Worcestershire sauce
- 1 tablespoon honey
- 1/2 teaspoon onion powder
- 1/2 teaspoon garlic powder
- 1/4 teaspoon black pepper
- 1/4 cup slivered almonds

Cooking Guidelines :

1) Preheat the oven to 175°F (80°C).
2) Cut the beef into thin strips, about 1/8 inch thick.
3) In a bowl, mix together the soy sauce, Worcestershire sauce, honey, onion powder, garlic powder, and black pepper.
4) Add the beef strips to the bowl and toss to coat them evenly with the marinade. Let the beef marinate for at least 30 minutes, or overnight in the fridge.
5) Spread the beef strips out in a single layer on a baking sheet lined with parchment paper.
6) Sprinkle the slivered almonds over the top of the beef strips.
7) Bake the beef jerky in the preheated oven for 4-6 hours, or until it is dry and chewy. Flip the beef strips over halfway through cooking to ensure even drying.
8) Once the beef jerky is done, remove it from the oven and let it cool completely before storing in an airtight container.

Chapter 2: Post-Op Diet Recipes (Phase 1: Clear Liquids)

The Post-Op Diet (Phase 1)

Following a strict diet after gastric sleeve surgery is essential to ensuring that your body heals correctly and preventing any problems. The first post-op diet typically lasts four to six weeks and is divided into four phases, each with its own set of Cooking Guidelines .

You'll be on a liquid diet for the first phase, which normally lasts one to two weeks. Your stomach will be less stressed as a result, and it will have more time to recover completely. You must drink clear liquids like water, broth, and gelatin without added sugar.

You may go to pureed meals in the second stage, which lasts for two to four weeks. At this stage, you should still refrain from eating solid meals, but you may start adding things like soft-boiled eggs, pureed veggies, and low-fat Greek yogurt.

Transitioning to soft foods is part of the third stage of the post-op diet, which normally lasts for two to four weeks. You'll start adding solid meals back into your diet at this point, but they must be soft and simple to digest. Fish that has been cooked through, canned fruit, and cooked veggies are a few examples of soft meals.

The maintenance phase, which begins around three months following surgery, is the last phase of the post-op diet. You may now begin to consume a more diversified diet, but you should still watch your portion sizes and stay away from anything that can make you feel sick.

Post-op 7 Days Meal Plan (Phase 1)

Day 1

Breakfast:

- 1 cup clear chicken broth
- 1 sugar-free gelatin cup

Snack:

- 1 cup of sugar-free popsicles

Lunch:

- 1 cup clear beef broth
- 1 cup sugar-free gelatin

Snack:

- 1 cup of sugar-free popsicles

Dinner:

- 1 cup clear vegetable broth
- 1 cup sugar-free gelatin

Snack:

- 1 cup of sugar-free popsicles

Day 2

Breakfast:

- 1 cup clear chicken broth
- 1 sugar-free gelatin cup

Snack:

- 1 cup of sugar-free popsicles

Lunch:

- 1 cup clear beef broth
- 1 cup sugar-free gelatin

Snack:

- 1 cup of sugar-free popsicles

Dinner:

- 1 cup clear vegetable broth
- 1 cup sugar-free gelatin

Snack:

- 1 cup of sugar-free popsicles

Day 3

Breakfast:

- 1 cup clear chicken broth
- 1 sugar-free gelatin cup

- 1 cup of sugar-free popsicles

Lunch:

- 1 cup clear beef broth
- 1 cup sugar-free gelatin

Snack:

- 1 cup of sugar-free popsicles

Dinner:

- 1 cup clear chicken broth with 1/2 cup strained tomato soup
- 1 sugar-free gelatin cup

Snack:

- 1 cup of sugar-free popsicles

Day 4

Breakfast:

- 1 cup clear chicken broth
- 1 sugar-free gelatin cup

Snack:

- 1 cup of sugar-free popsicles

Lunch:

- 1 cup clear vegetable broth
- 1 sugar-free gelatin cup

Snack:

- 1 cup of sugar-free popsicles

Dinner:

- 1 cup clear beef broth with 1/2 cup strained tomato soup
- 1 sugar-free gelatin cup

Snack:

- 1 cup of sugar-free popsicles

Day 5

Breakfast:

- 1 cup clear chicken broth
- 1 sugar-free gelatin cup

Snack:

- 1 cup of sugar-free popsicles

Lunch:

- 1 cup clear beef broth
- 1 sugar-free gelatin cup

Snack:

- 1 cup of sugar-free popsicles

Dinner:

- 1 cup clear vegetable broth with 1/2 cup strained chicken noodle soup
- 1 sugar-free gelatin cup

- 1 cup of sugar-free popsicles

Day 6

Breakfast:

- 1 cup clear chicken broth
- 1 sugar-free gelatin cup

Snack:

- 1 cup of sugar-free popsicles

Lunch:

- 1 cup clear beef broth
- 1 sugar-free gelatin cup

Snack:

- 1 cup of sugar-free popsicles

Dinner:

- 1 cup clear chicken broth with 1/2 cup strained vegetable soup
- 1 sugar-free gelatin cup

Snack:

- 1 cup of sugar-free popsicles

Day 7

- 1 cup clear chicken broth
- 1 sugar-free gelatin cup

Snack:

- 1 cup of sugar-free popsicles

Lunch:

- 1 cup clear vegetable broth
- 1 sugar-free gelatin cup

Snack:

- 1 cup of sugar-free popsicles

Dinner:

- 1 cup clear beef broth with 1/2 cup strained chicken noodle soup

Post- Op Diet Phase 1: Clear Liquid Recipes

BASIC CHICKEN BROTH

Ingredients:

- 1 whole chicken, cleaned and chopped into small pieces
- 1 onion, chopped
- 2 cloves of garlic, chopped
- 2 celery stalks, chopped

- 2 carrots, chopped
- 10 cups of water
- Salt and pepper to taste

Cooking Guidelines :

1) In a large pot, add the chicken, onion, garlic, celery, carrots, and water.
2) Bring the mixture to a boil over high heat.
3) Once boiling, reduce the heat to low and let simmer for 2-3 hours.
4) Strain the mixture through a fine mesh strainer.
5) Add salt and pepper to taste.
6) Serve hot.

LEMON AND GINGER CHICKEN BROTH:

Ingredients:

- 1 whole chicken, cleaned and chopped into small pieces
- 1 onion, chopped
- 2 cloves of garlic, chopped
- 2 celery stalks, chopped
- 2 carrots, chopped
- 10 cups of water
- 1 lemon, sliced
- 1-inch piece of fresh ginger, sliced
- Salt and pepper to taste

Cooking Guidelines :

1) In a large pot, add the chicken, onion, garlic, celery,

carrots, water, lemon, and ginger.

2) Bring the mixture to a boil over high heat.
3) Once boiling, reduce the heat to low and let simmer for 2-3 hours.
4) Strain the mixture through a fine mesh strainer.
5) Add salt and pepper to taste.
6) Serve hot.

SPICY CHICKEN BROTH

Ingredients:

- 1 whole chicken, cleaned and chopped into small pieces
- 1 onion, chopped
- 2 cloves of garlic, chopped
- 2 celery stalks, chopped
- 2 carrots, chopped
- 10 cups of water
- 1 jalapeno pepper, chopped
- 1 teaspoon of cumin
- Salt and pepper to taste

Cooking Guidelines :

1) In a large pot, add the chicken, onion, garlic, celery, carrots, water, jalapeno pepper, and cumin.
2) Bring the mixture to a boil over high heat.
3) Once boiling, reduce the heat to low and let simmer for 2-3 hours.
4) Strain the mixture through a fine mesh strainer.
5) Add salt and pepper to taste.

6) Serve hot.

CLEAR TOMATO SOUP

Ingredients:

- 2 lbs of fresh tomatoes, diced
- 2 cloves of garlic, minced
- 1 onion, chopped
- 2 cups of water
- Salt and pepper to taste
- 1 tablespoon of olive oil
- Fresh basil leaves for garnish

Cooking Guidelines :

1) In a large pot, heat the olive oil over medium heat.
2) Add the garlic and onion and cook until softened, about 5-7 minutes.
3) Add the diced tomatoes and cook for another 10-12 minutes, stirring occasionally.
4) Add the water and bring the mixture to a boil.
5) Reduce the heat to low and let simmer for 10-15 minutes.
6) Remove from heat and let cool for a few minutes.
7) Using an immersion blender, blend the mixture until smooth.
8) Strain the mixture through a fine mesh strainer to remove any seeds or skins.
9) Season with salt and pepper to taste.
10) Serve hot with fresh basil leaves for garnish.

SUGAR-FREE JELLO

Ingredients:

- 1 package of sugar-free Jello (any flavor)
- 2 cups of boiling water
- 2 cups of cold water

Cooking Guidelines :

1) In a large bowl, add the sugar-free Jello mix.
2) Add the boiling water to the bowl and stir until the Jello mix is completely dissolved.
3) Add the cold water to the bowl and stir until well combined.
4) Pour the mixture into individual serving cups or a large serving dish.
5) Refrigerate the Jello for at least 2 hours or until set.
6) Serve chilled.

COCONUT WATER

Ingredients:

- 1 young coconut
- Ice (optional)

Cooking Guidelines :

1) Using a cleaver or a large knife, carefully cut off the top of the young coconut.
2) Pour the coconut water into a glass or bottle.
3) Add ice, if desired.
4) Enjoy chilled.

VEGETABLE BROTH

Ingredients:

- 2 carrots, chopped
- 2 celery stalks, chopped
- 1 onion, chopped
- 4 cups of water
- Salt and pepper to taste
- 1 tablespoon of olive oil

Cooking Guidelines :

1) In a large pot, heat the olive oil over medium heat.
2) Add the chopped carrots, celery, and onion and cook until softened, about 5-7 minutes.
3) Add the water and bring the mixture to a boil.
4) Reduce the heat to low and let simmer for 20-30 minutes.
5) Remove from heat and let cool for a few minutes.
6) Using a fine mesh strainer, strain the mixture into another pot or container.
7) Discard the vegetables and season the broth with salt and pepper to taste.
8) Serve hot or store in the refrigerator or freezer for later use.

VANILLA ALMOND PROTEIN SHAKE

Ingredients:

- 1 scoop of vanilla protein powder (whey or plant-based)
- 1 cup of unsweetened almond milk
- 1/2 teaspoon of vanilla extract
- Ice cubes (optional)

Cooking Guidelines :

1) In a blender, combine the protein powder, almond milk, and vanilla extract.
2) Add ice cubes, if desired, and blend until smooth.
3) Serve chilled.

BERRY BLAST PROTEIN SMOOTHIE

Ingredients

- 1 scoop of berry-flavored protein powder (whey or plant-based)
- 1 cup of water
- 1 cup of mixed frozen berries (strawberries, blueberries, raspberries, etc.)
- Ice cubes (optional)

Cooking Guidelines :

1) In a blender, combine the protein powder, water, and mixed frozen berries.
2) Add ice cubes, if desired, and blend until smooth.
3) Serve chilled.

TROPICAL PROTEIN PUNCH

Ingredients

- 1 scoop of vanilla protein powder (whey or plant-based)
- 1 cup of coconut water
- 1/2 cup of frozen pineapple chunks
- Ice cubes (optional)

Cooking Guidelines :

1) In a blender, combine the protein powder, coconut water, and frozen pineapple chunks.
2) Add ice cubes, if desired, and blend until smooth.
3) Serve chilled.

APPLE JUICE

Ingredients:

- 4 medium apples (any variety)
- 4 cups of water
- 1 tablespoon of lemon juice
- Stevia or other zero-calorie sweetener to taste (optional)

Cooking Guidelines :

1) Wash and core the apples, then slice them into thin pieces.
2) In a large pot, combine the sliced apples, water, and lemon juice.
3) Bring the mixture to a boil over medium-high heat.

4) Reduce the heat to low and let simmer for 20-30 minutes, or until the apples are very soft.
5) Remove from heat and let cool for a few minutes.
6) Using a fine mesh strainer, strain the mixture into another pot or container.
7) Discard the apple pieces and season the juice with stevia or other zero-calorie sweetener to taste.
8) Serve chilled or at room temperature.

LEMON WATER

Ingredients:

- 1 lemon
- 4 cups of water
- Stevia or other zero-calorie sweetener to taste (optional)
- Ice cubes (optional)

Cooking Guidelines :

1) Slice the lemon into thin rounds.
2) In a large pitcher or container, combine the lemon slices and water.
3) Cover and let sit in the refrigerator for at least 30 minutes, or overnight.
4) Remove the lemon slices and add stevia or other zero-calorie sweetener to taste, if desired.
5) Serve over ice, if desired.

CLEAR CHICKEN OR BEEF BROTH WITH EGG DROP

Ingredients:

- 4 cups of clear chicken or beef broth
- 2 eggs
- 1 tablespoon of cornstarch
- 1 tablespoon of cold water
- Salt and pepper to taste

Cooking Guidelines :

1) In a small bowl, whisk together the cornstarch and cold water until smooth.
2) In a saucepan, heat the clear chicken or beef broth until simmering.
3) Slowly pour the cornstarch mixture into the broth while stirring constantly.
4) Continue to stir until the broth has thickened slightly.
5) In another bowl, beat the eggs until frothy.
6) Slowly pour the beaten eggs into the broth while stirring constantly, creating egg ribbons.
7) Cook for another minute, then remove from heat.
8) Season with salt and pepper to taste.
9) Serve hot.

WATERMELON JUICE

Ingredients:

- 4 cups of cubed watermelon

- 1/4 cup of water
- 1 tablespoon of lemon juice
- Stevia or other zero-calorie sweetener to taste (optional)
- Ice cubes (optional)

Cooking Guidelines :

1) In a blender, puree the watermelon and water until smooth.
2) Strain the puree through a fine mesh strainer, discarding any solids.
3) Add lemon juice and stevia or other zero-calorie sweetener to taste, if desired.
4) Serve chilled over ice, if desired.

Chapter 3: Post-Op Diet Recipes (Phase 2: Full Liquids)

Post-op Meal Plan (Phase 2)

Day 1:

Breakfast: Protein shake made with low-fat milk or soy milk

Snack: Sugar-free Jell-O or pudding

Lunch: Cream of mushroom soup (blended to a smooth consistency) with a side of Greek yogurt

Snack: Low-fat yogurt

Dinner: Tomato soup (blended to a smooth consistency) with a side of protein shake

Day 2:

Breakfast: Protein shake made with low-fat milk or soy milk

Snack: Low-fat cottage cheese

Lunch: Broccoli and cheese soup (blended to a smooth

consistency) with a side of Greek yogurt

Snack: Sugar-free popsicle

Dinner: Creamy chicken soup (blended to a smooth consistency) with a side of protein shake

Day 3:

Breakfast: Protein shake made with low-fat milk or soy milk

Snack: Low-fat Greek yogurt

Lunch: Creamy tomato soup (blended to a smooth consistency) with a side of sugar-free Jell-O

Snack: Low-fat cottage cheese

Dinner: Cream of chicken soup (blended to a smooth consistency) with a side of protein shake

Day 4:

Breakfast: Protein shake made with low-fat milk or soy milk

Snack: Low-fat Greek yogurt

Lunch: Creamy cauliflower soup (blended to a smooth consistency) with a side of sugar-free pudding

Snack: Low-fat cottage cheese

Dinner: Cream of mushroom soup (blended to a smooth consistency) with a side of protein shake

Day 5:

Breakfast: Protein shake made with low-fat milk or soy milk

Snack: Sugar-free Jell-O or pudding

Lunch: Creamy zucchini soup (blended to a smooth consistency) with a side of Greek yogurt

Snack: Low-fat cottage cheese

Dinner: Creamy tomato soup (blended to a smooth consistency) with a side of protein shake

Day 6:

Breakfast: Protein shake made with low-fat milk or soy milk

Snack: Low-fat Greek yogurt

Lunch: Cream of broccoli soup (blended to a smooth consistency) with a side of sugar-free popsicle

Snack: Low-fat cottage cheese

Dinner: Creamy chicken soup (blended to a smooth consistency) with a side of protein shake

Day 7:

Breakfast: Protein shake made with low-fat milk or soy milk

Snack: Sugar-free Jell-O or pudding

Lunch: Creamy tomato soup (blended to a smooth consistency) with a side of Greek yogurt

Snack: Low-fat cottage cheese

Dinner: Creamy mushroom soup (blended to a smooth consistency) with a side of protein shake

Post-Op Diet Phase 2: Full Liquid Recipes

CREAMY TOMATO SOUP WITH GREEK YOGURT

Ingredients:

- 1 can of crushed tomatoes
- 1 cup of low-sodium vegetable broth
- 1/2 cup of plain Greek yogurt
- 1 small onion, chopped
- 2 garlic cloves, minced
- 1 tablespoon of olive oil
- 1/4 teaspoon of dried thyme
- Salt and pepper to taste

Cooking Guidelines :

1) Heat olive oil in a saucepan over medium heat. Add onions and garlic and sauté for 2-3 minutes, or until onions are translucent.
2) Add crushed tomatoes, vegetable broth, thyme, salt, and pepper. Stir well and bring to a simmer.
3) Reduce heat to low and let the soup cook for 15-20 minutes, or until the flavors have melded together.
4) Remove from heat and let cool for a few minutes.
5) Transfer the soup to a blender or food processor and blend until smooth.
6) Return the soup to the saucepan and stir in the Greek yogurt.
7) Heat the soup on low heat for 2-3 minutes, or until warmed through.
8) Serve hot

CREAMY TOMATO SOUP WITH COCONUT MILK

Ingredients:

- 1 can of diced tomatoes
- 1 cup of low-sodium vegetable broth
- 1/2 cup of coconut milk
- 1 small onion, chopped
- 2 garlic cloves, minced
- 1 tablespoon of olive oil
- 1/4 teaspoon of dried basil
- Salt and pepper to taste

Cooking Guidelines :

1) Heat olive oil in a saucepan over medium heat. Add onions and garlic and sauté for 2-3 minutes, or until onions are translucent.
2) Add diced tomatoes, vegetable broth, basil, salt, and pepper. Stir well and bring to a simmer.
3) Reduce heat to low and let the soup cook for 15-20 minutes, or until the flavors have melded together.
4) Remove from heat and let cool for a few minutes.
5) Transfer the soup to a blender or food processor and blend until smooth.
6) Return the soup to the saucepan and stir in the coconut milk.
7) Heat the soup on low heat for 2-3 minutes, or until warmed through.
8) Serve hot

CHOCOLATE PROTEIN SHAKE

Ingredients:

- 1 scoop of chocolate protein powder (check for one that is low in sugar and carbs)
- 1 cup of unsweetened almond milk
- 1/2 frozen banana
- 1/2 tablespoon of unsweetened cocoa powder
- 1/2 teaspoon of vanilla extract
- 1-2 ice cubes

Cooking Guidelines :

1) Add all the ingredients to a blender.
2) Blend on high for 1-2 minutes, or until smooth and creamy.
3) If the shake is too thick, add a little more almond milk until you reach the desired consistency.
   Taste and adjust sweetness as needed. If you prefer a sweeter shake, you can add a low-calorie sweetener such as stevia or monk fruit.

CREAMY MASHED CAULIFLOWER

Ingredients:

- 1 head of cauliflower, cut into florets
- 1/4 cup of low-sodium chicken or vegetable broth
- 1/4 cup of unsweetened almond milk
- 2 tablespoons of unsalted butter
- 1 garlic clove, minced
- Salt and pepper to taste

Cooking Guidelines :

1) Bring a large pot of salted water to a boil. Add the

cauliflower florets and boil for 10-15 minutes, or until tender.
2) Drain the cauliflower and transfer it to a food processor.
3) Add the chicken or vegetable broth, almond milk, butter, garlic, salt, and pepper to the food processor.
4) Process the mixture until smooth and creamy.
5) Taste and adjust seasoning as needed.
6) Serve hot

VANILLA YOGURT SMOOTHIE

Ingredients:

- 1/2 cup of plain Greek yogurt
- 1/2 cup of unsweetened almond milk
- 1/2 frozen banana
- 1/2 teaspoon of vanilla extract
- 1-2 ice cubes
- Optional: low-calorie sweetener such as stevia or monk fruit, to taste

Cooking Guidelines :

1) Add all the ingredients to a blender.
2) Blend on high for 1-2 minutes, or until smooth and creamy.
3) If the smoothie is too thick, add a little more almond milk until you reach the desired consistency.
4) Taste and adjust sweetness as needed. If you prefer a sweeter smoothie, you can add a low-calorie sweetener such as stevia or monk fruit.

CREAMY CHICKEN SOUP

Ingredients:

- 1 pound boneless, skinless chicken breasts, cut into small pieces
- 4 cups of low-sodium chicken broth
- 1/2 cup of heavy cream
- 1/2 cup of unsweetened almond milk
- 1 tablespoon of olive oil
- 1 onion, chopped
- 2 garlic cloves, minced
- 2 celery stalks, chopped
- 2 carrots, peeled and chopped
- Salt and pepper to taste
- Optional: fresh herbs such as thyme or rosemary for garnish

Cooking Guidelines :

1) In a large pot, heat the olive oil over medium heat.
2) Add the onion and garlic and sauté for 2-3 minutes, or until fragrant.
3) Add the chicken and cook until browned on all sides.
4) Add the chicken broth, celery, and carrots to the pot.
5) Bring the mixture to a boil, then reduce the heat and simmer for 15-20 minutes, or until the vegetables are tender and the chicken is cooked through.
6) Stir in the heavy cream and almond milk, and heat the soup for a few minutes until it's hot but not boiling.
7) Taste and adjust seasoning as needed.
8) Serve hot and garnish with fresh herbs, if desired.

GREEN SMOOTHIE

Ingredients:

- 1 cup of unsweetened almond milk
- 1 cup of baby spinach
- 1/2 frozen banana
- 1/2 green apple, chopped
- 1/2 cucumber, chopped
- 1 tablespoon of chia seeds
- 1/2 teaspoon of honey (optional)

Cooking Guidelines :

1) Add all the ingredients to a blender.
2) Blend on high for 1-2 minutes, or until smooth and creamy.
3) If the smoothie is too thick, add a little more almond milk until you reach the desired consistency.
4) Taste and adjust sweetness as needed. If you prefer a sweeter smoothie, you can add a little honey.

CREAM OF BROCCOLI SOUP

Ingredients:

- 1 head of broccoli, chopped into small florets
- 4 cups of low-sodium chicken or vegetable broth
- 1/2 cup of heavy cream
- 1/2 cup of unsweetened almond milk
- 1 tablespoon of olive oil
- 1 onion, chopped

- 2 garlic cloves, minced
- Salt and pepper to taste
- Optional: grated parmesan cheese for garnish

Cooking Guidelines :

1) In a large pot, heat the olive oil over medium heat.
2) Add the onion and garlic and sauté for 2-3 minutes, or until fragrant.
3) Add the broccoli and broth to the pot.
4) Bring the mixture to a boil, then reduce the heat and simmer for 15-20 minutes, or until the broccoli is tender.
5) Using an immersion blender or transferring the soup to a blender, blend until smooth.
6) Stir in the heavy cream and almond milk, and heat the soup for a few minutes until it's hot but not boiling.
7) Taste and adjust seasoning as needed.
8) Serve hot and garnish with grated parmesan cheese, if desired.

BLUEBERRY PROTEIN SMOOTHIE

Ingredients:

- 1 cup of unsweetened almond milk
- 1/2 cup of frozen blueberries
- 1 scoop of vanilla protein powder (whey, pea, or soy-based)
- 1 tablespoon of chia seeds
- 1/2 teaspoon of honey (optional)

Cooking Guidelines :

1) Add all the ingredients to a blender.
2) Blend on high for 1-2 minutes, or until smooth and creamy.
3) If the smoothie is too thick, add a little more almond milk until you reach the desired consistency.
4) Taste and adjust sweetness as needed. If you prefer a sweeter smoothie, you can add a little honey.

CREAMY CARROT SOUP

Ingredients:

- 1 pound of carrots, peeled and chopped
- 1 onion, chopped
- 2 garlic cloves, minced
- 4 cups of low-sodium chicken or vegetable broth
- 1/2 cup of heavy cream
- 1/2 cup of unsweetened almond milk
- 1 tablespoon of olive oil
- Salt and pepper to taste
- Optional: chopped fresh parsley for garnish

Cooking Guidelines :

1) In a large pot, heat the olive oil over medium heat.
2) Add the onion and garlic and sauté for 2-3 minutes, or until fragrant.
3) Add the chopped carrots and broth to the pot.
4) Bring the mixture to a boil, then reduce the heat and simmer for 20-25 minutes, or until the carrots are tender.
5) Using an immersion blender or transferring the soup

to a blender, blend until smooth.

6) Stir in the heavy cream and almond milk, and heat the soup for a few minutes until it's hot but not boiling.
7) Taste and adjust seasoning as needed.
8) Serve hot and garnish with chopped fresh parsley, if desired.

PEANUT BUTTER BANANA SMOOTHIE

Ingredients:

- 1 ripe banana, sliced
- 1 tablespoon of peanut butter (natural, no added sugar)
- 1 scoop of vanilla protein powder (whey, pea, or soy-based)
- 1 cup of unsweetened almond milk
- 1/2 teaspoon of cinnamon (optional)

Cooking Guidelines :

1) Add all the ingredients to a blender.
2) Blend on high for 1-2 minutes, or until smooth and creamy.
3) If the smoothie is too thick, add a little more almond milk until you reach the desired consistency.
4) Taste and adjust sweetness as needed. If you prefer a sweeter smoothie, you can add a little honey or a few drops of liquid stevia.

Chapter 4: Post-Op Diet Recipes (Phase 3: Soft Foods)

Day 1:

Breakfast: Greek yogurt with pureed fruit and a sprinkle of granola.

Snack: Protein shake.

Lunch: Pureed vegetable soup with soft crackers.

Snack: Cottage cheese with pureed fruit.

Dinner: Soft scrambled eggs with pureed vegetables.

Day 2:

Breakfast: Oatmeal with pureed fruit and a sprinkle of cinnamon.

Snack: Protein shake.

Lunch: Pureed chicken and vegetable stew.

Snack: Greek yogurt with pureed fruit.

Dinner: Pureed lentil soup with soft crackers.

Day 3:

Breakfast: Scrambled eggs with pureed vegetables and a side of fruit.

Snack: Protein shake.

Lunch: Soft tuna salad with avocado and pureed vegetables.

Snack: Cottage cheese with pureed fruit.

Dinner: Pureed beef and vegetable stew.

Day 4:

Breakfast: Protein pancake with pureed fruit and a sprinkle of nuts.

Snack: Protein shake.

Lunch: Pureed cauliflower and cheese soup with soft crackers.

Snack: Greek yogurt with pureed fruit.

Dinner: Pureed salmon and vegetable stew.

Day 5:

Breakfast: Scrambled eggs with pureed vegetables and a side of fruit.

Snack: Protein shake.

Lunch: Pureed chicken and mushroom soup with soft crackers.

Snack: Cottage cheese with pureed fruit.

Dinner: Pureed beef and vegetable casserole.

Day 6:

Breakfast: Protein waffles with pureed fruit and a sprinkle of nuts.

Snack: Protein shake.

Lunch: Soft turkey meatloaf with pureed vegetables.

Snack: Greek yogurt with pureed fruit.

Dinner: Pureed vegetable lasagna.

Day 7:

Breakfast: Omelets with pureed vegetables and a side of fruit.

Snack: Protein shake.

Lunch: Pureed mushroom and barley soup with soft crackers.

Snack: Cottage cheese with pureed fruit.

Dinner: Pureed chicken and vegetable curry.

Post-Op Diet Phase 3: Soft Food Recipes

BASIC CREAMY CAULIFLOWER SOUP

Ingredients:

- 1 large head cauliflower, chopped
- 1 onion, chopped
- 2 cloves garlic, minced
- 3 cups low-sodium chicken or vegetable broth
- 1 cup unsweetened almond milk
- Salt and pepper, to taste
- Chopped fresh parsley, for garnish (optional)

Cooking Guidelines :

1) In a large pot, sauté onion and garlic until tender.
2) Add cauliflower and broth. Bring to a boil, then reduce heat and simmer until cauliflower is very tender.
3) Use an immersion blender or transfer to a blender to puree the soup until smooth.
4) Add almond milk and stir until heated through.
5) Season with salt and pepper to taste.
6) Garnish with chopped parsley if desired.

CREAMY CAULIFLOWER AND BROCCOLI SOUP

Ingredients:

- 1 head cauliflower, chopped
- 1 head broccoli, chopped
- 1 onion, chopped
- 2 cloves garlic, minced
- 3 cups low-sodium chicken or vegetable broth

- 1 cup unsweetened almond milk
- Salt and pepper, to taste
- Chopped fresh chives, for garnish (optional)

Cooking Guidelines :

1) In a large pot, sauté onion and garlic until tender.
2) Add cauliflower, broccoli, and broth. Bring to a boil, then reduce heat and simmer until vegetables are very tender.
3) Use an immersion blender or transfer to a blender to puree the soup until smooth.
4) Add almond milk and stir until heated through.
5) Season with salt and pepper to taste.
6) Garnish with chopped chives if desired.

SPICY CREAMY CAULIFLOWER SOUP

Ingredients:

- 1 head cauliflower, chopped
- 1 onion, chopped
- 2 cloves garlic, minced
- 3 cups low-sodium chicken or vegetable broth
- 1/2 cup unsweetened almond milk
- 1/2 teaspoon smoked paprika
- 1/2 teaspoon cumin
- 1/4 teaspoon cayenne pepper
- Salt and pepper, to taste
- Chopped fresh cilantro, for garnish (optional)

Cooking Guidelines :

1) In a large pot, sauté onion and garlic until tender.
2) Add cauliflower and broth. Bring to a boil, then reduce heat and simmer until cauliflower is very tender.
3) Use an immersion blender or transfer to a blender to puree the soup until smooth.
4) Add almond milk and spices, and stir until heated through.
5) Season with salt and pepper to taste.
6) Garnish with chopped cilantro if desired.

BASIC MASHED SWEET POTATOES

Ingredients:

- 2 large sweet potatoes, peeled and chopped
- 1/4 cup unsweetened almond milk
- 1 tablespoon unsalted butter
- Salt and pepper, to taste
- Chopped fresh parsley, for garnish (optional)

Cooking Guidelines :

1) Boil sweet potatoes until very tender, about 20 minutes.
2) Drain the potatoes and add almond milk, butter, salt, and pepper.
3) Mash with a potato masher or immersion blender until smooth.
4) Garnish with chopped parsley if desired.

SPICY MASHED SWEET POTATOES

Ingredients:

- 2 large sweet potatoes, peeled and chopped
- 1/4 cup unsweetened almond milk
- 1 tablespoon unsalted butter
- 1/4 teaspoon cumin
- 1/4 teaspoon chili powder
- Salt and pepper, to taste
- Chopped fresh cilantro, for garnish (optional)

Cooking Guidelines :

1) Boil sweet potatoes until very tender, about 20 minutes.
2) Drain the potatoes and add almond milk, butter, cumin, chili powder, salt, and pepper.
3) Mash with a potato masher or immersion blender until smooth.
4) Garnish with chopped cilantro if desired.

SWEET AND SAVORY MASHED SWEET POTATOES

Ingredients:

- 2 large sweet potatoes, peeled and chopped
- 1/4 cup unsweetened almond milk
- 1 tablespoon unsalted butter
- 1 tablespoon maple syrup
- 1/4 teaspoon cinnamon
- Salt and pepper, to taste

- Chopped pecans, for garnish (optional)

Cooking Guidelines :

1) Boil sweet potatoes until very tender, about 20 minutes.
2) Drain the potatoes and add almond milk, butter, maple syrup, cinnamon, salt, and pepper.
3) Mash with a potato masher or immersion blender until smooth.
4) Garnish with chopped pecans if desired.

LENTIL AND VEGETABLE STEW

Ingredients:

- 1 tablespoon olive oil
- 1 small onion, chopped
- 2 cloves garlic, minced
- 2 carrots, peeled and chopped
- 2 stalks celery, chopped
- 1/2 cup dry lentils, rinsed and drained
- 1 can diced tomatoes, undrained
- 1 cup low-sodium vegetable broth
- 1/2 teaspoon dried thyme
- Salt and pepper, to taste
- Chopped fresh parsley, for garnish (optional)

Cooking Guidelines :

1) Heat olive oil in a large pot over medium heat. Add onion and garlic and sauté until onion is translucent, about 5 minutes.

2) Add carrots and celery and sauté for another 5
   minutes.
3) Add lentils, diced tomatoes, vegetable broth, thyme,
   salt, and pepper. Stir to combine.
4) Bring the mixture to a boil, then reduce heat to low
   and cover the pot. Simmer for 30-40 minutes, or until
   lentils are tender.
5) Use an immersion blender to blend the stew to a
   desired consistency or alternatively you can mash it
   up using a potato masher.
6) Garnish with chopped parsley if desired.

TUNA SALAD

Ingredients:

- 1 can of tuna in water, drained
- 2 tablespoons plain Greek yogurt
- 1 tablespoon low-fat mayonnaise
- 1 celery stalk, chopped
- 1 tablespoon red onion, chopped
- Salt and pepper, to taste
- Optional add-ins: chopped pickles, diced apples,
  chopped walnuts

Cooking Guidelines :

1) In a small mixing bowl, combine the drained tuna,
   Greek yogurt, and low-fat mayonnaise. Mix well.
2) Add the chopped celery and red onion, and any
   optional add-ins you desire.
3) Season with salt and pepper to taste, and mix until all
   ingredients are evenly distributed.

4) Serve the tuna salad on top of a bed of lettuce, on top
of whole grain bread, or wrapped in lettuce leaves.

SCRAMBLED EGGS

Ingredients:

- 2 large eggs
- 1 tablespoon unsweetened almond milk or low-fat
  milk
- Salt and pepper, to taste
- 1 teaspoon olive oil or non-stick cooking spray
- Optional add-ins: diced vegetables such as bell
  peppers, onions, or spinach, diced lean ham or turkey,
  shredded low-fat cheese

Cooking Guidelines :

1) In a small mixing bowl, whisk together the eggs,
   almond milk, and salt and pepper until well
   combined.
2) Heat a non-stick skillet over medium heat and add the
   olive oil or non-stick cooking spray.
3) Add any optional add-ins and sauté until the
   vegetables are tender or the ham/turkey is lightly
   browned.
4) Pour in the egg mixture and use a spatula to gently
   scramble the eggs until cooked to your desired level of
   doneness.
5) Serve hot

CHICKEN AND VEGETABLE STIR FRY

Ingredients:

- 4 oz boneless, skinless chicken breast, cut into bite-sized pieces
- 1 tablespoon low-sodium soy sauce
- 1 tablespoon cornstarch
- 1 tablespoon olive oil
- 1/2 cup sliced onion
- 1/2 cup sliced bell peppers
- 1/2 cup sliced zucchini
- 1/2 cup sliced mushrooms
- 1 garlic clove, minced
- Salt and pepper, to taste

Cooking Guidelines :

1) In a small mixing bowl, whisk together the soy sauce and cornstarch until well combined.
2) Add the chicken pieces to the bowl and toss to coat evenly.
3) Heat the olive oil in a non-stick skillet over medium-high heat.
4) Add the onion and sauté until softened, about 2-3 minutes.
5) Add the bell peppers, zucchini, mushrooms, and garlic and sauté for another 2-3 minutes until the vegetables are tender.
6) Push the vegetables to the side of the skillet and add the chicken to the center.
7) Cook the chicken for 2-3 minutes until lightly browned, then stir in the vegetables.
8) Season with salt and pepper to taste and serve hot.

COTTAGE CHEESE AND FRUIT SALAD

Ingredients:

- 1/2 cup low-fat cottage cheese
- 1/2 cup mixed fruit (such as berries, sliced kiwi, or diced melon)
- 1 tablespoon chopped nuts (such as almonds or walnuts)
- 1 teaspoon honey (optional)

Cooking Guidelines :

1) In a small mixing bowl, combine the cottage cheese and mixed fruit.
2) Add the chopped nuts and mix until evenly distributed.
3) Drizzle with honey, if desired.
4) Serve cold

GREEK YOGURT PARFAIT

Ingredients:

- 1/2 cup plain non-fat Greek yogurt
- 1/2 cup mixed fruit (such as berries, sliced kiwi, or diced mango)
- 1 tablespoon chopped nuts (such as almonds or pecans)

- 1 teaspoon honey (optional)

Cooking Guidelines :

1) In a small serving dish or jar, layer the Greek yogurt, mixed fruit, and chopped nuts.
2) Drizzle with honey, if desired.
3) Repeat the layering process until all ingredients are used up.
4) Serve cold

BUTTERNUT SQUASH SOUP

Ingredients:

- 1 small butternut squash, peeled and diced
- 1 small onion, diced
- 1 garlic clove, minced
- 1 tablespoon olive oil
- 2 cups low-sodium chicken or vegetable broth
- Salt and pepper, to taste

Cooking Guidelines :

1) In a large pot, heat the olive oil over medium heat.
2) Add the onion and garlic and sauté until softened, about 2-3 minutes.
3) Add the diced butternut squash and sauté for another 2-3 minutes.
4) Pour in the broth and bring to a boil.
5) Reduce the heat and simmer for 20-25 minutes, until the squash is tender.
6) Use an immersion blender or transfer the mixture to a

blender and puree until smooth.
7) Season with salt and pepper to taste.
8) Serve hot

SOFT TACOS

Ingredients:

- 4 small corn tortillas
- 4 ounces cooked and shredded chicken breast
- 1/4 cup chopped lettuce
- 1/4 cup chopped tomato
- 1 tablespoon chopped onion
- 1 tablespoon chopped cilantro
- 1/2 avocado, diced
- 1/4 cup low-fat shredded cheese
- Salt and pepper, to taste
- Salsa and lime wedges, for serving (optional)

Cooking Guidelines :

1) Warm the corn tortillas in a microwave or on a griddle until pliable.
2) Divide the shredded chicken, lettuce, tomato, onion, cilantro, and avocado among the tortillas.
3) Sprinkle each taco with shredded cheese.
4) Season with salt and pepper to taste.
5) Fold the tortillas in half to form tacos.
6) Serve hot with salsa and lime wedges, if desired.

Chapter 5: Post-Op Diet Recipes (Phase 4: Regular Diet)

Day 1:

Breakfast: Scrambled eggs with diced tomatoes and spinach, and a slice of whole-grain toast.

Snack: Greek yogurt with sliced strawberries and a tablespoon of honey.

Lunch: Grilled chicken breast with mixed greens salad, cherry tomatoes, cucumber, and a vinaigrette dressing.

Snack: Sliced apple with almond butter.

Dinner: Baked salmon with roasted asparagus and quinoa.

Day 2:

Breakfast: Protein smoothie made with unsweetened almond milk, frozen berries, and vanilla protein powder.

Snack: Low-fat string cheese with a handful of grapes.

Lunch: Turkey chili with kidney beans, diced tomatoes, and green chilies.

Snack: Roasted chickpeas.

Dinner: Grilled sirloin steak with roasted Brussels sprouts and sweet potato wedges.

Day 3:

Breakfast: Cottage cheese with sliced peaches and a sprinkle of cinnamon.

Snack: Hard-boiled egg with a handful of baby carrots.

Lunch: Tuna salad with mixed greens, cherry tomatoes, and a vinaigrette dressing.

Snack: Roasted edamame.

Dinner: Grilled shrimp skewers with grilled zucchini and brown rice.

Day 4:

Breakfast: Avocado toast with a poached egg and a side of fresh fruit.

Snack: Apple slices with peanut butter.

Lunch: Grilled chicken Caesar salad with romaine lettuce, cherry tomatoes, and a light Caesar dressing.

Snack: Low-fat cottage cheese with a handful of blueberries.

Dinner: Baked chicken breast with steamed broccoli and cauliflower mash.

Day 5:

Breakfast: Omelet with diced bell peppers, mushrooms, and shredded cheddar cheese.

Snack: Low-fat Greek yogurt with sliced almonds and a drizzle of honey.

Lunch: Grilled portobello mushroom burger with mixed greens, tomato, and avocado.

Snack: Baby carrots with hummus.

Dinner: Baked cod with roasted vegetables and a quinoa salad.

Day 6:

Breakfast: Protein pancakes with fresh berries and a drizzle of sugar-free syrup.

Snack: Hard-boiled egg with a handful of cherry tomatoes.

Lunch: Grilled turkey burger with mixed greens, tomato, and avocado.

Snack: Roasted pumpkin seeds.

Dinner: Grilled chicken kebabs with grilled peppers and onions and a side of brown rice.

Day 7:

Breakfast: Greek yogurt parfait with granola and mixed

berries.

Snack: Low-fat string cheese with a handful of raspberries.

Lunch: Grilled salmon with mixed greens, cherry tomatoes, and a vinaigrette dressing.

Snack: Baby carrots with ranch dressing.

Dinner: Grilled flank steak with grilled zucchini and a side of quinoa salad.

Post-Op Diet Phase 4: Regular Diet Recipes

LEMON AND HERB BAKED CHICKEN BREAST:

Ingredients:

- 4 boneless, skinless chicken breasts
- 2 tbsp. olive oil
- 2 tbsp. lemon juice
- 1 tbsp. dried oregano
- 1 tbsp. dried thyme
- Salt and pepper to taste

Cooking Guidelines :

1) Preheat your oven to 375°F.
2) In a small bowl, whisk together the olive oil, lemon juice, oregano, thyme, salt, and pepper.
3) Place the chicken breasts in a baking dish and brush them with the lemon and herb mixture.
4) Bake the chicken breasts in the preheated oven for 25-

30 minutes, or until they reach an internal
temperature of 165°F.

5) Remove the chicken from the oven and let it rest for 5-10 minutes before serving.

PESTO AND PARMESAN BAKED CHICKEN BREAST

Ingredients:

- 4 boneless, skinless chicken breasts
- 2 tbsp. olive oil
- 2 tbsp. pesto sauce
- 2 tbsp. grated Parmesan cheese
- Salt and pepper to taste

Cooking Guidelines :

1) Preheat your oven to 375°F.
2) In a small bowl, mix together the olive oil, pesto sauce, grated Parmesan cheese, salt, and pepper.
3) Place the chicken breasts in a baking dish and brush them with the pesto and Parmesan mixture.
4) Bake the chicken breasts in the preheated oven for 25-30 minutes, or until they reach an internal temperature of 165°F.
5) Remove the chicken from the oven and let it rest for 5-10 minutes before serving.

LEMON AND HERB GRILLED TILAPIA

Ingredients:

- 4 tilapia fillets
- 2 tbsp. olive oil
- 2 tbsp. lemon juice
- 1 tbsp. dried oregano
- 1 tbsp. dried thyme
- Salt and pepper to taste

Cooking Guidelines :

1) Preheat your grill to medium-high heat.
2) In a small bowl, whisk together the olive oil, lemon juice, oregano, thyme, salt, and pepper.
3) Brush the tilapia fillets with the lemon and herb mixture.
4) Grill the tilapia fillets for 3-4 minutes per side, or until they are cooked through and flaky.
5) Remove the tilapia from the grill and let it rest for a few minutes before serving.

CHILI LIME GRILLED SALMON

Ingredients:

- 4 salmon fillets
- 2 tbsp. olive oil
- 2 tbsp. lime juice
- 1 tbsp. chili powder
- Salt and pepper to taste

Cooking Guidelines :

1) Preheat your grill to medium-high heat.
2) In a small bowl, whisk together the olive oil, lime
   juice, chili powder, salt, and pepper.
3) Brush the salmon fillets with the chili lime mixture.
4) Grill the salmon fillets for 4-5 minutes per side, or
   until they are cooked through and flaky.
5) Remove the salmon from the grill and let it rest for a
   few minutes before serving.

BEEF AND VEGETABLE STIR FRY

Ingredients:

- 1 lb. lean beef, sliced into thin strips
- 2 tbsp. olive oil
- 2 cups mixed vegetables (broccoli, bell peppers,
  carrots, onions, etc.)
- 1 tbsp. low-sodium soy sauce
- 1 tbsp. cornstarch
- 1 tbsp. water
- Salt and pepper to taste

Cooking Guidelines :

1) Heat the olive oil in a large skillet or wok over high
   heat.
2) Add the beef strips to the skillet and cook for 2-3
   minutes, or until they are browned on all sides.
3) Add the mixed vegetables to the skillet and stir-fry for
   2-3 minutes, or until they are tender-crisp.
4) In a small bowl, whisk together the soy sauce,
   cornstarch, water, salt, and pepper.
5) Add the soy sauce mixture to the skillet and stir-fry

for another 1-2 minutes, or until the sauce thickens
and coats the beef and vegetables.

6) Remove the skillet from the heat and serve the beef
and vegetable stir-fry hot.

TURKEY CHILI

Ingredients:

- 1 lb. ground turkey
- 1 tbsp. olive oil
- 1 onion, chopped
- 2 bell peppers, chopped
- 2 cloves garlic, minced
- 1 can diced tomatoes (14.5 oz)
- 1 can kidney beans, drained and rinsed (15 oz)
- 1 can black beans, drained and rinsed (15 oz)
- 2 tbsp. chili powder
- 1 tsp. ground cumin
- Salt and pepper to taste

Cooking Guidelines :

1) Heat the olive oil in a large pot or Dutch oven over
medium heat.
2) Add the ground turkey to the pot and cook until it is
browned and cooked through, breaking it up with a
wooden spoon as it cooks.
3) Add the chopped onion, bell peppers, and garlic to the
pot and sauté until the vegetables are tender.
4) Add the diced tomatoes, kidney beans, black beans,
chili powder, cumin, salt, and pepper to the pot and

stir to combine.

5) Bring the chili to a simmer and let it cook for 15-20 minutes, or until the flavors have melded together and the vegetables are tender.

6) Serve the turkey chili hot, garnished with your favorite toppings such as shredded cheese, chopped cilantro, or a dollop of Greek yogurt.

QUINOA SALAD

Ingredients:

- 1 cup quinoa, rinsed
- 2 cups water
- 1/4 cup chopped red onion
- 1/4 cup chopped fresh parsley
- 1/4 cup chopped fresh mint
- 1/4 cup chopped fresh cilantro
- 1/4 cup chopped cherry tomatoes
- 1/4 cup chopped cucumber
- 1/4 cup chopped bell pepper
- 2 tbsp. olive oil
- 2 tbsp. fresh lemon juice
- Salt and pepper to taste

Cooking Guidelines :

1) Combine the quinoa and water in a medium saucepan and bring to a boil over high heat.

2) Reduce the heat to low and simmer, covered, for 15-20 minutes, or until the quinoa is tender and the water has been absorbed.

3) Fluff the quinoa with a fork and transfer it to a large bowl.
4) Add the red onion, parsley, mint, cilantro, cherry tomatoes, cucumber, and bell pepper to the bowl and toss to combine.
5) In a small bowl, whisk together the olive oil, lemon juice, salt, and pepper.
6) Drizzle the dressing over the quinoa salad and toss to coat.
7) Serve the quinoa salad chilled or at room temperature, garnished with additional fresh herbs if desired.

ZUCCHINI NOODLES WITH MEATBALLS

Ingredients:

For the meatballs:

- 1 lb. lean ground beef or turkey
- 1/4 cup almond flour
- 1 egg
- 1/4 cup grated parmesan cheese
- 2 cloves garlic, minced
- 2 tbsp. chopped fresh parsley
- 1 tsp. dried oregano
- Salt and pepper to taste

For the zucchini noodles:

- 4 medium zucchinis, spiraled

- 2 tbsp. olive oil
- 2 cloves garlic, minced
- Salt and pepper to taste

Cooking Guidelines :

1) Preheat the oven to 375°F.
2) In a large bowl, mix together the ground beef or turkey, almond flour, egg, parmesan cheese, garlic, parsley, oregano, salt, and pepper until well combined.
3) Form the mixture into small meatballs, about 1-2 inches in diameter.
4) Place the meatballs on a baking sheet lined with parchment paper and bake for 15-20 minutes, or until cooked through.
5) While the meatballs are baking, prepare the zucchini noodles. Heat the olive oil in a large skillet over medium heat.
6) Add the minced garlic to the skillet and sauté for 30 seconds, or until fragrant.
7) Add the spiraled zucchini noodles to the skillet and cook for 2-3 minutes, or until tender but still slightly firm.
8) Season the zucchini noodles with salt and pepper to taste.
9) Serve the zucchini noodles topped with the meatballs.

TURKEY AND VEGGIE BURGER

Ingredients:

- 1 lb. lean ground turkey

- 1 cup grated zucchini
- 1/4 cup chopped fresh parsley
- 1/4 cup chopped fresh cilantro
- 2 cloves garlic, minced
- 1/2 tsp. ground cumin
- Salt and pepper to taste
- 4 whole wheat buns
- Optional toppings: lettuce, tomato, onion, avocado

Cooking Guidelines :

1) In a large bowl, mix together the ground turkey, grated zucchini, parsley, cilantro, garlic, cumin, salt, and pepper until well combined.
2) Divide the mixture into 4 equal portions and form each portion into a patty.
3) Heat a nonstick skillet over medium-high heat and add the patties to the skillet.
4) Cook the patties for 4-5 minutes on each side, or until cooked through and browned.
5) Toast the whole wheat buns in a toaster or oven.
6) Place each turkey and veggie burger patty on a toasted bun and top with optional toppings if desired.

BAKED SALMON WITH ROASTED VEGETABLES

Ingredients:

- 4 salmon fillets (4-6 oz. each)
- 2 tbsp. olive oil
- 2 tbsp. lemon juice
- 2 cloves garlic, minced

- Salt and pepper to taste
- 2 cups chopped mixed vegetables (such as broccoli, cauliflower, and bell peppers)

Cooking Guidelines :

1) Preheat the oven to 400°F.
2) In a small bowl, whisk together the olive oil, lemon juice, garlic, salt, and pepper.
3) Place the salmon fillets in a baking dish and brush them with the olive oil mixture.
4) Arrange the chopped vegetables around the salmon fillets in the baking dish.
5) Brush the vegetables with the remaining olive oil mixture.
6) Bake the salmon and vegetables in the preheated oven for 12-15 minutes, or until the salmon is cooked through and the vegetables are tender.

GREEK SALAD WITH GRILLED CHICKEN

Ingredients:

- 2 boneless, skinless chicken breasts (4-6 oz. each)
- 1 tbsp. olive oil
- 1 tbsp. lemon juice
- 1 clove garlic, minced
- Salt and pepper to taste
- 4 cups chopped mixed greens
- 1 cup chopped cucumber
- 1 cup cherry tomatoes, halved
- 1/2 cup chopped red onion

* 1/2 cup crumbled feta cheese
* 1/4 cup pitted Kalamata olives
* 2 tbsp. chopped fresh parsley
* 2 tbsp. chopped fresh dill
* Optional dressing: 2 tbsp. olive oil and 1 tbsp. red wine vinegar

Cooking Guidelines :

1) Preheat a grill or grill pan to medium-high heat.
2) In a small bowl, whisk together the olive oil, lemon juice, garlic, salt, and pepper.
3) Brush the chicken breasts with the olive oil mixture.
4) Grill the chicken breasts for 5-6 minutes on each side, or until cooked through.
5) Remove the chicken from the grill and let it rest for 5 minutes before slicing.
6) In a large bowl, mix together the mixed greens, cucumber, cherry tomatoes, red onion, feta cheese, Kalamata olives, parsley, and dill.
7) Top the salad with the sliced grilled chicken.
8) Drizzle the salad with the optional olive oil and red wine vinegar dressing, if desired.

STUFFED BELL PEPPERS

Ingredients:

* 4 bell peppers, halved and seeded
* 1 lb. lean ground turkey
* 1/2 cup cooked quinoa
* 1/2 cup chopped onion

- 1/2 cup chopped celery
- 1/2 cup chopped carrots
- 1 clove garlic, minced
- 1 tsp. dried oregano
- Salt and pepper to taste
- 1 cup canned crushed tomatoes
- 1/4 cup chopped fresh parsley
- 1/4 cup shredded mozzarella cheese

Cooking Guidelines :

1) Preheat the oven to 375°F.
2) In a large skillet, cook the ground turkey over medium heat until browned.
3) Add the onion, celery, carrots, garlic, oregano, salt, and pepper to the skillet and cook until the vegetables are tender.
4) Add the cooked quinoa and crushed tomatoes to the skillet and stir until well combined.
5) Stuff the bell pepper halves with the turkey and quinoa mixture.
6) Place the stuffed bell peppers in a baking dish and bake in the preheated oven for 25-30 minutes, or until the peppers are tender and the filling is heated through.
7) Remove the stuffed bell peppers from the oven and sprinkle the shredded mozzarella cheese on top of each pepper.
8) Return the peppers to the oven and bake for an additional 5-10 minutes, or until the cheese is melted and bubbly.

Final Thoughts

Congrats on making the decision to seek gastric sleeve bariatric surgery as a first step in improving your health. It's a courageous and noble choice, and I'm here to give you some closing advice and suggestions for your adventure.

Remember that the surgery itself is simply a minor part of the process as you begin this new chapter in your life. After the procedure, the hard work starts when you decide to adopt new, healthy habits that will help you achieve your weight reduction objectives.

Your nutrition will be one of the most crucial components of your recovery after surgery. I'm happy to suggest this gastric sleeve bariatric diet cookbook to you as a useful tool. This cookbook is filled with delicious and healthful dishes that have been specially created to fulfill the requirements of patients who have undergone weight loss. You'll discover everything you need to support your body's healing process and maintain a healthy weight with its focus on protein-rich foods, low-carb alternatives, and simple-to-digest meals.

But, this book is made up of more than simply a list of recipes. It serves as a reminder that food can be nutritious and pleasant as well as a guide to good eating. Remember to keep your attention on the constructive changes you're making in your life while you flip through its pages and test out new recipes. You should be happy with yourself for taking this crucial step, and don't forget to recognize your accomplishments as you go.

Keep in mind that every action, no matter how tiny, counts as progress. Hence, keep moving whether you're just getting started or well along. Keep working toward your objectives, have faith in the process, and never forget your immense potential.

I wish you luck on your path and am certain that you will lead the healthy, fulfilling life you deserve with the aid of this cookbook and your own willpower.

ABOUT THE AUTHOR

Aashvi Dhingra is an India born woman who currently resides in the United States. Aashvi has always been passionate about food and nutrition, which led her to pursue a career as a Registered Dietitian. Aashvi earned her Bachelor's degree in Nutrition and Dietetics from a prestigious university in India, and later received her Master's degree in Nutrition Science from a renowned university in the United States.

Aashvi's journey as a dietitian began in India, where she worked in various clinical and community settings. During her time in India, Aashvi developed a keen interest in the intersection between food, culture, and health. She conducted several research studies on the impact of traditional Indian diets on health outcomes, which earned her recognition and awards from various academic and research organizations.

In the United States, Aashvi has worked as a clinical dietitian in a hospital setting, where she has helped patients with various health conditions achieve their nutrition goals. Aashvi has also worked with several community organizations to promote healthy eating habits and improve access to nutritious foods.

Apart from her professional work as a dietitian, Aashvi is an avid home cook who loves experimenting with new recipes and flavors. She believes that cooking is a creative and therapeutic process that brings people together and fosters cultural exchange. Aashvi often shares her recipes and cooking tips on her social media platforms and has gained a significant following.

Aashvi's multicultural background and experience as a dietitian have shaped her approach to food and nutrition. She believes that a healthy and balanced diet should be personalized to an individual's cultural background, preferences, and lifestyle. Aashvi also emphasizes the importance of food education and empowering individuals to make informed choices about their diet.

Through her work as a dietitian and her passion for cooking, Aashvi hopes to inspire others to prioritize their health and well-being through food. She also aims to promote cultural understanding and celebrate the diversity of cuisines and culinary traditions around the world.

In her free time, Aashvi enjoys traveling, hiking, and exploring new restaurants and food markets. She is also an avid reader and enjoys learning about new topics related to food, culture, and health.

9 7 9 8 3 9 1 2 1 9 6 0 6